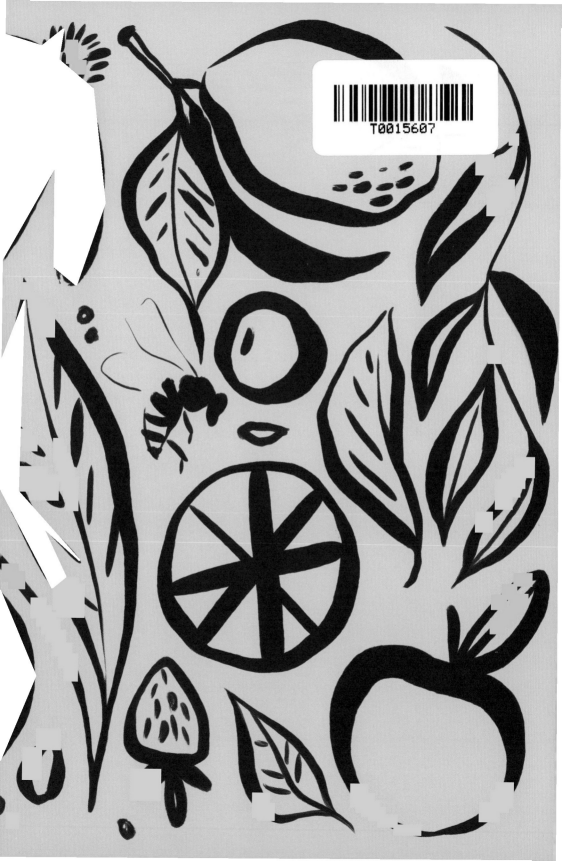

T0015607

RESTORE

Lizzie King

Ancient Remedies from
the Modern Kitchen

CONTENTS

INTRODUCTION

RESTORE: NOUN

To bring back; reinstate a previous custom or return someone or something to their original condition or way of being.

–

In today's landscape, staying well and in optimal health is often secondary to simply getting on until something is broken. Our medical system is primed to treat acute issues, to cure diseases and save lives. But it is our responsibility to think holistically and to maintain our good health, re-establishing a respect for the intrinsic power of nature, and reinstating this inherent knowledge, helping to restore our planet as we do so.

I am passionate about empowering people to take back control in optimising their own health and wellbeing by using simple and effective natural ingredients that are readily available in the world around us and that work in harmony with our bodies and the environment – ingredients that are low cost, accessible to everyone and non-toxic to the planet.

Our world is glittering with natural ingredients. Botanicals have been used for millennia as remedies without damaging side effects for us or our planet, but in recent times have been overlooked in favour of commercial, convenient and synthetic products, and so the health of our ecosystem and its biodiversity have been impacted.

I want to make it easy, enjoyable and motivating to get back to these ingredients from nature; to keep you and your home replete with simple, natural recipes and remedies for everyday life that are free from unnecessary harsh chemicals; that reduce the impact on our over-burdened planet as well as on your purse; to boost our resilience and combat the rigours of modern living.

Originally created for me and my family to thrive in optimal health, these are the ways I've found that we can enlist the natural world to help – a holistic approach from the inside out and the outside in. From tonics that aid sleep and balms for anxiety, syrups for avoiding the seasonal lurgies or coping with a sick bug, to fizzing bath bombs, edible face masks and lickable kitchen sprays, they have proven their efficacy time and time again through my lovely community on my blog 'Lizzie Loves Healthy' and benefit our whole selves – health for now and future-proofing us all.

This is a compendium of my findings. I hope you fall in love with making them, eating them, healing from them and giving them to others.

'The art of healing comes from nature, not from the physician. Therefore the physician must start from nature, with an open mind.'
– PARACELSUS, 16TH-CENTURY SWISS PHYSICIAN

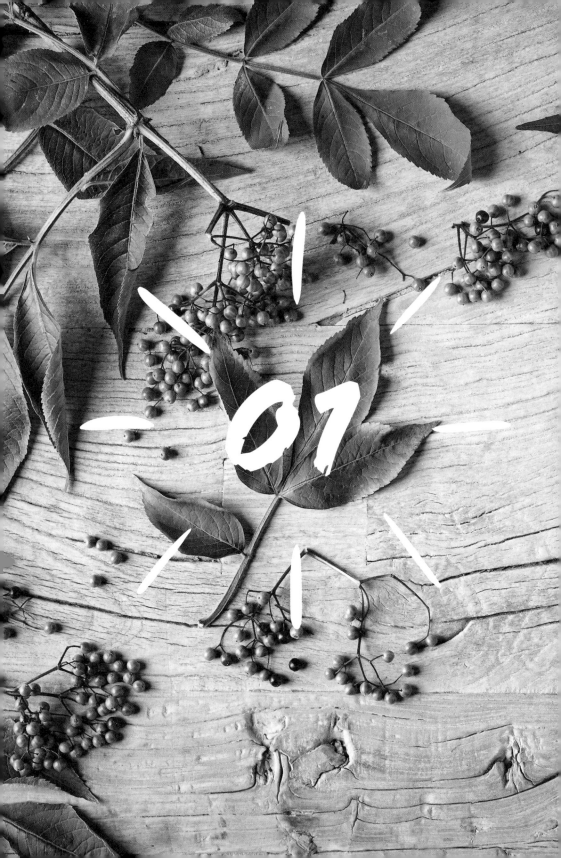

HEAL

As a cook and nutritional health coach, I always had my eye on
how to maximise the nourishing ingredients in anything I made
for my family and shared with others on my blog. And from there
I came to realise the power and popularity of targeting nutrients
for specific situations, seasons or concerns.

The highly prized purple plant polyphenols from the elderberry
were my initiation into making my own tonic to assuage those
ever-present winter lurgies that we can't seem to avoid. The
simplicity of making it, coupled with the successful outcomes,
buoyed me up and made me look at further ways of preventing
ill health by healing our bodies before or at the onset of
common health ailments. To prevent and protect.

These are remedies to aid and assist you at times of knocks,
coughs, aches and grazes. Helping and healing in a gentle,
natural way that works with your ever-capable system to
restore you to your best.

ELDERBERRY SYRUP

Elderberries were my first ever foray into plucking ingredients from the hedgerows to bubble up for my family's health. The elderberry has always been prized for its antiviral and antimicrobial properties – so much so that there was a global shortage recently. I had been pouring the sticky elderberry derivative into my children for years when I realised I could make a better version at home with more fresh antioxidants. The dark colour of the *Sambucus nigra*, providing the precious anthocyanins, is where all the antiviral properties lie. This eventually led to my BE WELL remedy, but this purple goodness is where it all started. Spoon it out in winter and notice how the cough and cold season just doesn't hit you in the same way.

INGREDIENTS

~ 150g (5oz/1 cup) elderberries, rinsed (or 2 elderberry and echinacea tea bags – I love Pukka)

~ 2.5cm (1in) ginger root, peeled and thinly sliced

~ 1 tsp ground cinnamon

~ pinch of ground cloves

~ zest and juice of ½ orange

~ 750ml (25fl oz/3 cups) boiling water

~ juice of ½ lemon

~ 90g (3¼oz/¼ cup) raw honey

MAKES
About 1 litre
(34fl oz/4 cups)

METHOD

Put the elderberries (or the teabags) in a small saucepan and add the ginger, cinnamon, cloves and orange zest. Pour over the water, then place over a low heat and simmer gently for 20–30 minutes until it has reduced to roughly half the volume. Leave to cool slightly, then stir in the orange, lemon juices and the honey.

Strain and pour into a glass jar or bottle.

Storage: Store in the jar in the refrigerator for up to 3 months.

Dose: 2 teaspoons per child per day for children aged 1–2; 1 tablespoon per child per day for children over 2; 1 tablespoon 3–4 times a day for adults.

NOTE: Honey is not suitable for children under 1 year.

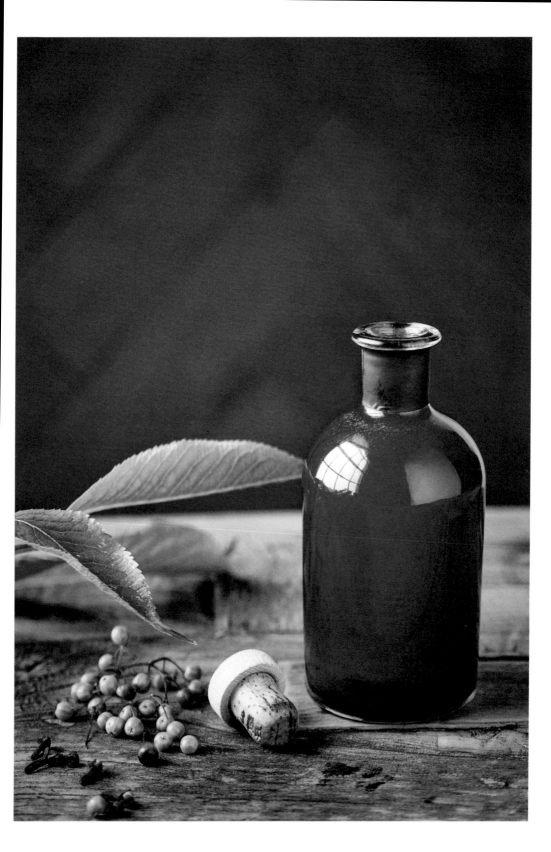

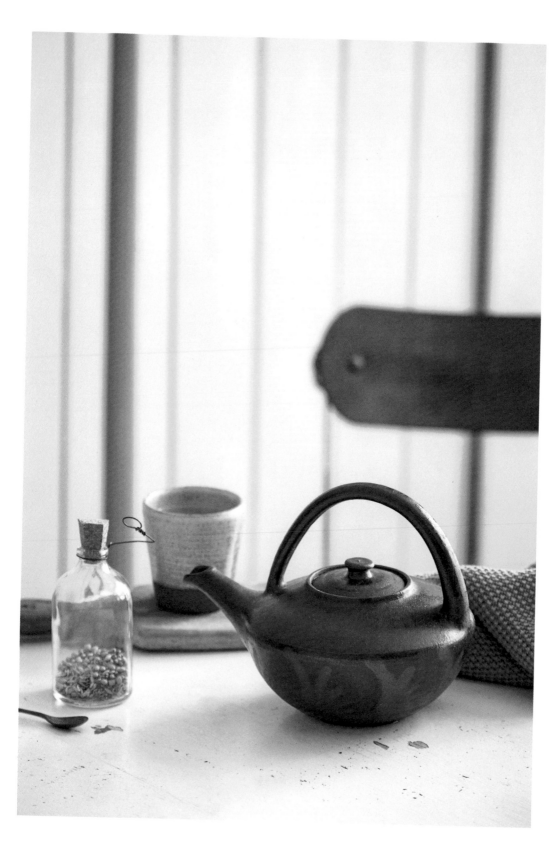

CUMIN & FENNEL SEED SICKNESS & DIGESTION INFUSION

A staple in India, eating fennel seeds after a meal both aids digestion and helps combat bloating, and this combination is the perfect evening drink if you're feeling full, nauseous, have heartburn or just need a digestif after a large meal.

INGREDIENTS

~ 1 tsp cumin seeds

~ 1 tsp fennel seeds

~ 1 tsp coriander seeds

~ 400ml (13fl oz/generous 1½ cups) boiling water

METHOD

Add the seeds to a teapot and pour in the boiling water. Allow to steep for 5–10 minutes, then pour and sip slowly.

Storage: Make fresh as required.

Dose: Sip after meals or as required.

MAKES
About 400ml
(13fl oz/generous
1½ cups)

VINEGAR & BROWN PAPER POULTICE BRUISE & SPRAIN RELIEF

It turns out there was truth to the rhyme and Jack was onto something, as applying a vinegar poultice has been shown to be effective for helping with bruises and swelling. The acidic vinegar increases the blood supply to the surface of the skin and thus speeds up the healing, brings down the swelling and helps the bruising dissipate. Ice and arnica are great here, too, but if you don't have ice available (many people don't like it anyway!), this is one to try.

INGREDIENTS

~ 120ml (4fl oz/½ cup) apple cider vinegar

~ 250ml (8½fl oz/1 cup) warm water

~ strips of sturdy brown paper or cloth, sized according to the area of the wound

METHOD

Mix the liquids together in a large bowl or bucket and soak each strip of paper. Apply to the wounded area, then wrap with a cloth. Leave on for 30 minutes, then wipe the area with clean water.

Storage: Make fresh as required.

Dose: Repeat twice a day until the swelling and bruising have gone down.

MAKES
About 350ml
(12¼fl oz/1½ cups)

SOOTHING ITCH-RELIEF OAT BATH SOAK

Oats possess some valuable skin-nourishing properties and include the chemical constituents saponins, which have a foamy soap-like quality. A natural cleanser as well as an exfoliant and emollient, they can calm when there is inflammation and irritation. This soak is useful for eczema flare-ups, chicken pox spots and psoriasis – a simple way of nurturing our largest organ.

INGREDIENTS

~ 300g (10½oz/3 cups) rolled oats

~ 1 pair of tights

~ 1 hot bath

MAKES
Enough for
one bath

METHOD

Pour the oats into an old pair of thinnish tights and tie a knot at the end.

Hang the oat sausage from one of the taps in the bath and turn on both taps so that the water filters through the oats as it runs into the bath.

Soak in the bath for 20–30 minutes to relieve redness and itching. Pat dry gently.

Storage: Make fresh as required.

Dose: Use daily as needed.

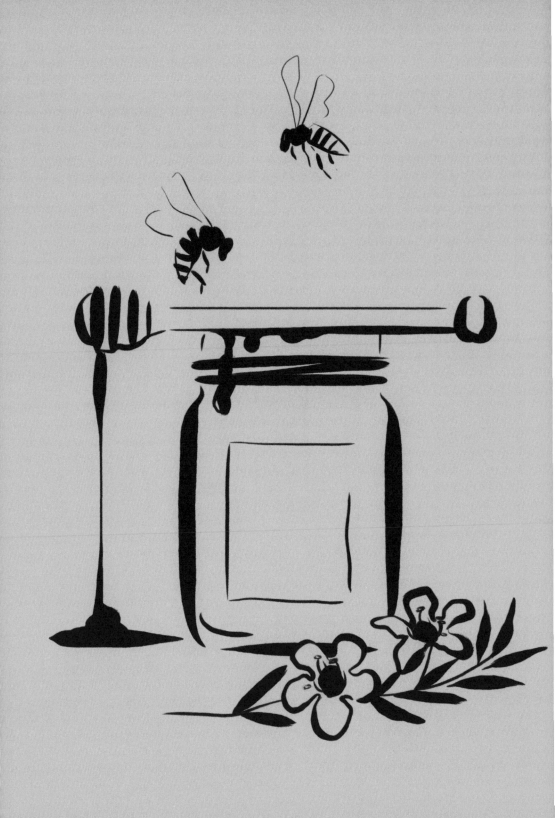

SPOTLIGHT ON
HONEY

One of the most ancient and universal ingredients used for healing, honey is a celebrated natural product of sustainability, seasonality and palatability. Honeybees were producing their sweet golden liquid for 14 million years, undisturbed, foraging nectar from the flowers and storing the sticky biproduct in their hives, until the first humans realised, about 10,000 years ago, that they made more than they needed. The Egyptians exploited the antibacterial potential of honey and they enjoyed it liberally: in their food and drink, to preserve bodies and medicinally as a salve for wounds. Ancient Greek physicians, traditional Chinese medicine and Ayurveda all cite honey in early texts, noting the symbiotic relationship between man and bee and the countless healing applications it has, from topical balms for wounds or eye infections to ingesting for stomach ailments, coughs or asthma. The Qur'an has a piece dedicated to honeybees and their produce, calling it 'a drink of varying colours, containing healing for mankind'.

High in polyphenols, which makes it a great antioxidant, honey also possesses natural antiviral, antibacterial, antifungal and antimicrobial properties, which is why it is a remedy with such a wide variety of functions. Today's shop-bought honey has often been through a process of heat treatment, which degrades the peroxide activity and enzymes and alters those distinctive floral flavours and aromas before reaching the jar, so look for raw, unpasteurised honey. And check the label for TA (Total Activity), measuring the levels of antimicrobial activity scored from 1 to 20; 10+ is considered a substantial amount.

Studies recently caught up with folkloric wisdom and proved that honey is the most effective treatment for coughs, resulting in the NHS changing their guidelines in 2018 to recommend honey for coughs in place of antibiotics – a testament to just how well it works.

TURMERIC & HONEY ANTIBACTERIAL COLD & FLU RELIEF

Called 'golden honey' in Ayurveda, this combination of honey and the active curcumin ingredient in this prized root is dubbed 'nature's antibiotic' for the powerful antibacterial, antimicrobial and anti-inflammatory properties it possesses. Make a batch as the weather starts to cool and you'll have it ready if you feel the start of a cold.

INGREDIENTS

~ 100g (3½oz/scant ⅓ cup) raw honey

~ 1 tbsp ground turmeric

~ grind of black pepper

METHOD

Pour the honey into a clean, sterilised jar. Add the turmeric powder and a single grind of black pepper and stir well to combine.

Serve neat, ½ teaspoon onto the tongue and let it dissolve, then repeat as needed.

Storage: Keeps for up to 1 month.

Dose: Take ½ teaspoon on the first day, then increase to 1 teaspoon a day.

NOTE: Honey is not suitable for children under 1 year.

MAKES
About 75ml
(2½fl oz/scant
⅓ cup)

GINGER & HONEY COUGH SYRUP

The honey base here means you can more easily serve up raw and potent ginger to younger children who might not otherwise manage the fiery flavour. Research has shown that ginger can be effective in reducing the pain from tonsillitis as well as sore throats. This is a no-cook remedy that can be ready almost instantly when needed.

INGREDIENTS

~ 7.5cm (3in) ginger root, peeled and minced

~ 1 tbsp raw honey

MAKES
One serving

METHOD

Pass the ginger through a sieve (fine mesh strainer) – it's simpler than juicing in this quantity – which should yield 1 teaspoon of ginger juice. Mix the ginger juice with the honey and serve the full tablespoon onto the tongue, swallowing slowly as it dissolves.

TIP: For those who dare – slowly chewing a raw clove of garlic is a fabulous throat saver.

Storage: Makes fresh as required.

Dose: Repeat as needed.

NOTE: Honey is not suitable for children under 1 year.

CINNAMON SUGAR-BALANCING ALMOND BUTTER

Cinnamon is a warm, fragrant addition to a creamy nut butter that upgrades most snacks – a slice of apple, a banana or a piece of toast – but it also helps insulin regulation and thus balancing blood sugar. This is decreed by my youngest as 'the best nut butter ever tasted'.

INGREDIENTS

~ 300g (10½oz/2 cups) almonds, skin on

~ 1 tbsp coconut oil

~ pinch of sea salt flakes

~ 2 tbsp ground cinnamon

METHOD

Preheat the oven to 180°C (350°F/gas 4). Spread the nuts over a large, lined baking tray with the coconut oil, salt and cinnamon. Roast for 10 minutes – the smells will hint at the creation to come – shake the tray, turning the nuts, and roast for a further 3–5 minutes, watching they don't catch.

Remove from the oven and leave to cool for a moment.

Tip into the bowl of a high-powered blender or food processor and blend on low for 1–2 minutes, scraping down the nuts from the side as you go. Once a paste, blend on high for a further 3–5 minutes.

Transfer to an airtight jar.

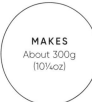

MAKES
About 300g
(10¼oz)

Storage: Keep in a jar in the refrigerator for up to a month.

Dose: Spread onto toast, crackers, apple slices or use as a dip.

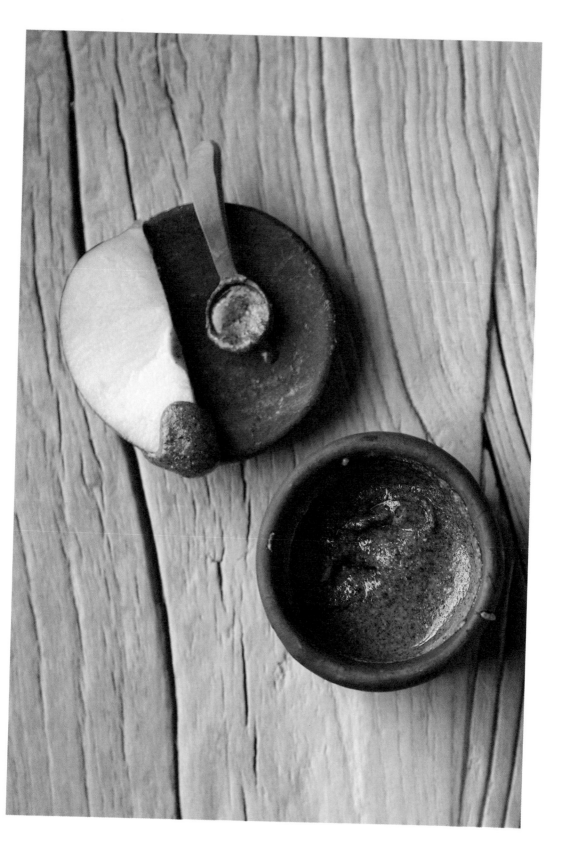

EARACHE VINEGAR REMEDY

As a child I spent many hours in the ENT department at the hospital and rode through many an antibiotic cycle as a result. My son took on my ear infection propensity, but I attempted to steer us from endless antibiotics when I could and found these ear drops used at the very first signs were often effective at quelling the onset.

INGREDIENTS

~ 2 tbsp apple cider vinegar

~ 2 tbsp cooled boiled water

METHOD

Mix the two liquids together in a clean cup. With the person lying on their side with the affected ear facing up, soak a cotton wool ball in the liquid, place it in the ear and leave to sit for 5 minutes. Remove the cotton wool and let any residual liquid drain out. Pat dry with a towel.

Storage: Make fresh as required.

Dose: Use a couple of times a day as needed.

MAKES
One application

FLU-BUSTING CHICKEN & GINGER BROTH

A steaming bowl of golden goodness is just what you need when your immune system is below par, you're recovering from something or you're hit by a bout of cold or flu. This combines the antiviral power of ginger with some sinus-clearing flavours in a bone broth to nourish and heal. Keep portions of this in the freezer to heat up whenever needed. You can perk it up by throwing in some fresh herbs as you warm it through and serve with freshly sliced mushrooms.

INGREDIENTS

~ 1 whole chicken

~ 2 celery stalks, roughly chopped

~ 1 large carrot, roughly chopped

~ 10cm (4in) ginger root, peeled and chopped

~ 1 tbsp black peppercorns

~ 2 tsp sea salt flakes

~ 1 onion, quartered

~ 1 bunch of parsley, rosemary and thyme, tied together, plus extra to serve

~ filtered water, as needed

~ salt and freshly ground black pepper, to taste

METHOD

Starting with the chicken, place all the ingredients into a large saucepan, tucking the chopped veg in and behind, then cover completely with filtered water. Bring to the boil over a high heat, then reduce to a simmer, covering partially with a lid. Skim off any froth that forms, then let it very gently simmer away for at least 3 hours (up to 12 hours). Keep an eye on the water level and top it up with boiling water every hour or two.

Turn off the heat and remove the chicken from the pan, taking the flesh from it with a fork and reserving. Strain off and discard the vegetables and bones.

Pour the soup into bowls, adding the cooked chicken slices and fresh herbs and seasoning with salt and pepper.

Storage: Cool any remaining soup, then store in glass bottles in the refrigerator or fill ice-cube trays and freeze.

Dose: Serve as often as you like.

TIP: Use a teaspoon to scrape the peel off the ginger.

MAKES
About 3 litres
(105fl oz/12 cups)

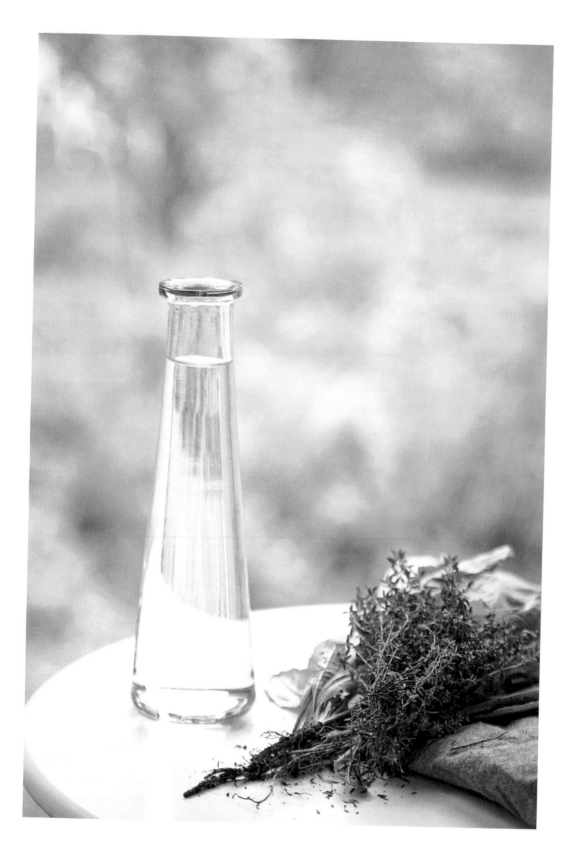

DANDELION & THYME GOUT RELIEF TONIC

The name dandelion – from *dent de lion* or lion's tooth – derives from the shape of the leaf. The root has commonly been used as a liver and digestive tonic, while thyme is well known as an antioxidant with anti-ageing properties. This combination is a pick-me-up for low days and the morning after. It has been used as a gout remedy, too.

INGREDIENTS

~ 2 tsp cleaned and chopped dandelion root

~ 2 tsp chopped thyme

~ 800ml (28fl oz/3½ cups) filtered water

METHOD

Place all the ingredients in a saucepan and bring to the boil. Reduce the heat, cover and simmer for 15–20 minutes. Leave to cool, then store in an airtight jar in the refrigerator. Take once a day.

Storage: Keep in the refrigerator for up to 1 month.

Dose: 100ml (3½fl oz/scant ½ cup) shots as needed.

MAKES
About 750ml
(25fl oz/3 cups)

TONSILLITIS COCONUT & MANGO POPSICLES

Tonsillitis and other very sore throats or inflammation from coughing can mean that swallowing anything is extremely painful, and the appetite dramatically decreases at a time when nutrients are needed most to combat the infection. Lollies are often accepted willingly, and as soothing as they are to swallow, these ingredients are also designed to help shore up the immune system.

INGREDIENTS

~ 200ml (7fl oz/scant 1 cup) coconut milk

~ 200g (7oz) frozen mango

~ 1 kiwi, peeled

~ 2 tbsp cashews

METHOD

Blend all the ingredients in a high-speed blender, then pour into lolly moulds. Place in the freezer until solid, at least 2 hours, depending on size.

Storage: Freeze for up to 12 months.

Dose: Serve as often as you like.

MAKES
About 4 lollies, depending on moulds

BERRY IMMUNE SLUSHIE

A fruity slushie when throats are sore is a happy delivery mechanism for important immune support such as vitamin C, antioxidants and anthocyanins. For those who choose not to have dairy, they also make a nice alternative to smoothies.

INGREDIENTS

~ 200g (7oz/1¼ cups) frozen berries

~ 100ml (3½fl oz/scant ½ cup) fresh orange juice

~ 2.5cm (1in) ginger root, peeled and chopped

~ 1 tbsp Elderberry Syrup (page 8)

~ 100g (3½oz) ice

METHOD

Add all the ingredients, except the ice, to a blender and blend until smooth. Add the ice and pulse until the consistency is chunky but drinkable. Pour into a tall glass and enjoy.

Storage: Make fresh as required.

Dose: Serve as often as you like.

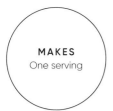

MAKES
One serving

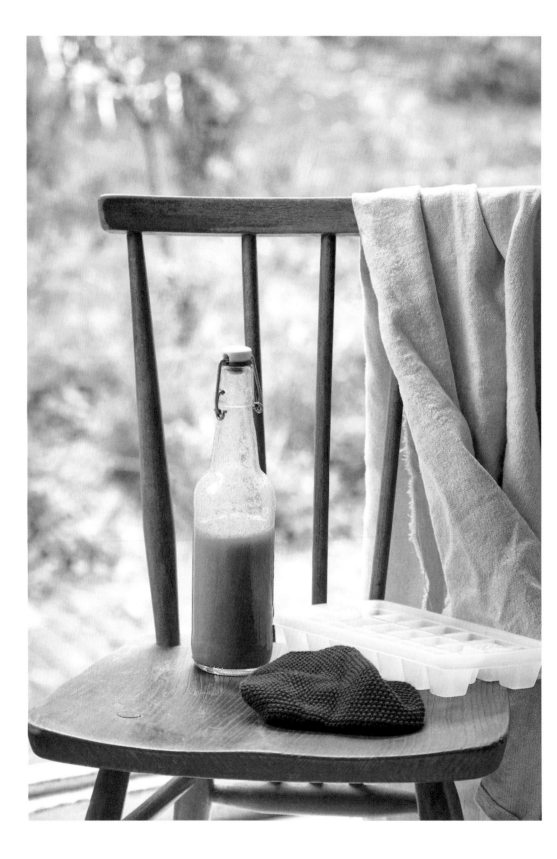

COLD RECOVERY TURMERIC, GINGER & LEMON INFUSION

This tonic can be kept in the freezer in ice-cube trays, so that when you need it you can just add one to hot water and go, with none of the prep. Turmeric is an intense orange-coloured root that has been prized for its powerful healing properties by Ayurveda for centuries. Recent studies have confirmed its cancer-protective and antiviral properties. Along with ginger, vitamin C-rich citrus and throat-soothing honey, this is a fiercely combative combination that helps me through coughs, colds and flu.

INGREDIENTS

~ 7.5cm (3in) turmeric root, peeled

~ 7.5cm (3in) ginger root, peeled

~ 1 lemon, peeled

~ 1 orange, peeled

~ 200ml (7fl oz/scant 1 cup) hot water

~ 2 tbsp raw honey

~ grind of black pepper

METHOD

In a juicer, juice together the turmeric, ginger, orange and lemon to yield about 200ml (7fl oz/scant 1 cup) of juice.

To use it immediatley, put 1–2 tablespoons in a cup and add the hot water, stirring in the honey to taste and adding a grind of pepper.

To save it for later, pour the juice into ice-cube trays and freeze, then pop into a freezer bag (it'll take up less space). Add the water, honey and pepper to administer.

Storage: Freeze for up to 12 months.

Dose: Repeat 2–4 times a day as needed.

NOTE: Honey is not suitable for children under 1 year.

MAKES
About 200ml
(7fl oz/scant
1 cup)

COCONUT OIL GRAZE BALM

Little cuts and grazes are the staple of small children and pets, so having a tube of antiseptic cream in the cupboard is always handy. Having seen the healing beauty of simple coconut oil, I used it as an all-purpose balm. The caprylic and lauric acid content means it has that magical triumvirate of antibacterial, antiviral and antifungal properties, making it a fabulous solution for all wounds, cuts, scrapes and grazes for man or beast. It has a high vitamin E content to promote skin healing, too, and one study has even shown that it is effective for bacteria that are antibiotic-resistant.

INGREDIENTS

~ 1 tsp coconut oil, at room temperature

METHOD

Smooth the oil over the affected area 2–3 times a day until healed. If using on pets or small children, you may want to apply to a cotton wool pad and cover with a bandage to keep them from licking, touching or irritating the area.

Storage: Store coconut oil in the refrigerator, then leave to warm to room temperature before using.

Dose: Apply 2–3 times a day.

MAKES
One application

MINT & FENNEL INDIGESTION TINCTURE

The word tincture has a beautiful ring of the apothecary about it, and it denotes something made by soaking herbs in alcohol in order to extract the active plant constituents. Tinctures are therefore more potent than a tea or infusion and are more robust, lasting up to two years. Stomach-settling mint and fennel make a lovely combination and this keeps in the medicine cabinet for any nausea, heartburn and indigestion woes that may come your way.

INGREDIENTS

~ 50g (1¾oz) mint leaves

~ 50g (1¾oz) fennel seeds

~ 100ml (3½fl oz/scant ½ cup) boiling water

~ 500ml (17fl oz/2 cups) alcohol (see Tip)

METHOD

Add the mint and fennel to a 1 litre (34fl oz/4 cup) jar or bottle, pour over the boiling water, making sure it covers the herbs, then add the alcohol. Label and place the lid on until cooled. Shake and place on a dark shelf, then leave to distil for 4–6 weeks, shaking every so often.

Strain through a muslin (cheesecloth) and funnel into a brown glass bottle.

Storage: Store in a dark bottle in a cool place for up to 2 years.

Dose: For adults, take 1 teaspoon in a glass of water at times of nausea or indigestion. For children under 18, take 10–20 drops in water.

TIP: 35–40% budget vodka is ideal.

MAKES
About 600ml
(20fl oz/2½ cups)

COLD & FLU DECONGESTING SOAK

Baths are fairly critical to my wellbeing. I relish my hot bath in the evening, as an escape, a sanctuary and as a point of total relaxation and switching off. I relied on them when pregnant and feeling cumbersome, and when the children were tiny it marked the blissful punctuation from manic days to the calm of the evening. I still have a hot bath on most nights. I light a calming candle and sometimes read a book, but often just rest. So I thought a nurturing, healing addition to a bath would be something to look forward to when feeling under the weather.

Long, hot baths when you're feeling blocked up, full of flu or aching are both a luxurious treat and do you some good; they are the comfort food of downtime. And by using the combination of respiratory-easing herbs and oils, you are helping your sinuses by clearing them out and melting away headaches with pine-scented aromatics. Or try adding lavender oil in place of eucalyptus for a soothing evening soak.

INGREDIENTS

~ 225g (8oz/1 cup) Epsom salts

~ 1 tsp bicarbonate of soda (baking soda)

~ 1 tsp almond oil

~ 10 drops of eucalyptus essential oil

METHOD

Tip the salts and soda into a mixing bowl or jug, drop the oils on top and mix well, then transfer to a jar for storage.

Storage: Stays fresh up to 3 months.

Dose: Add a handful to a hot bath every day for a long medicinal soak.

TIP: A simple way to ease sinus congestion is to hang eucalyptus (dried or fresh) in the shower, and as the steam percolates through the leaves, the oil's compounds are released and the respiratory benefits can be appreciated.

MAKES
About 250g
(9oz/generous
1 cup)

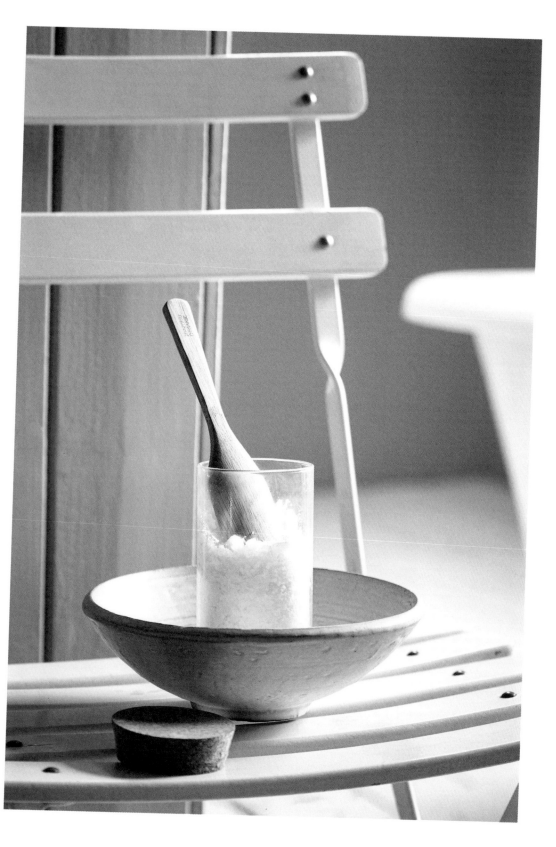

ANTI-INFLAMMATORY BLACK PEPPER & TURMERIC MORNING TONIC

A brilliant way to set yourself up for the day, or an effective curb to feeling low, I use this as a catch-all tonic for health. The power of turmeric is unlocked by the alkaloid, piperine, found in black pepper, as well as the fat content in the coconut oil, so combining them here maximises the efficacy of this anti-inflammatory root. The active compound, curcumin, is thus more bio-available, and as well as helping combat free radicals in our body, it stimulates our own production of antioxidants.

INGREDIENTS

~ 1 carrot, peeled and roughly chopped

~ juice of 1 orange

~ juice of 1 lemon

~ pinch of black pepper

~ 1 tbsp peeled and minced turmeric root

~ 1 tsp coconut oil

METHOD

Place all the ingredients into a powerful blender and pulse until liquidised. Drink immediately.

Storage: Make fresh as required.

Dose: Serve daily.

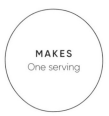

MAKES
One serving

ANTIVIRAL CASHEW & PARSLEY PESTO

A great way to get most people (and children) to eat raw garlic,
I serve this as is traditional, with pasta, but I love it spooned onto soups,
warm potatoes or spread on toast as a luxurious snack to enjoy, as well
as contributing a kick to our immune systems.

INGREDIENTS

~ 30g (1oz/1 cup) basil leaves, chopped

~ 15g (½oz/½ cup) parsley, chopped

~ 2 garlic cloves, peeled and minced

~ 50g (1¾oz/⅓ cup) cashews

~ 50g (1¾oz/⅓ cup) pine nuts

~ zest of ½ lemon

~ juice of 1 lemon

~ 100ml (3½fl oz/scant ½ cup) extra virgin olive oil

~ 1 tsp sea salt flakes

~ pinch of black pepper

METHOD

Place the herbs and garlic into the bowl of a food processor, add the nuts, seeds, lemon zest and juice, then drizzle in the oil as you pulse to blend, gradually increasing the olive oil until you have a pasta sauce consistency. Season to taste with salt and pepper.

Serve raw on top of soups, toast and salads, or stir into cooked pasta and top with Parmesan.

Storage: Make fresh as required or you can store in a jar under oil in the refrigerator for 3–4 days.

Dose: Serve as often as you like.

MAKES
About 300g
(10½oz)

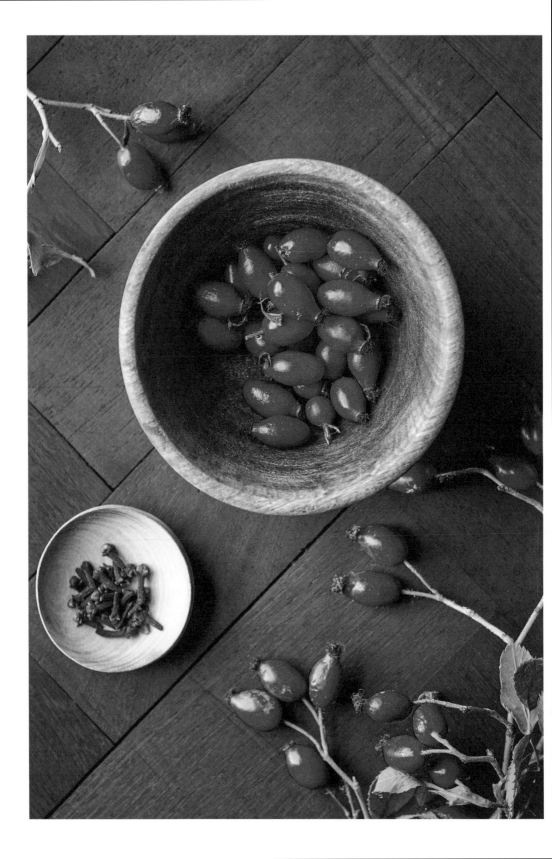

ROSEHIP & CLOVE WINTER SYRUP

A lovely way to ward off the winter lurgies using your hedgerows as medicine.
These crimson fruits are a seasonal winner, appearing just as the temperature dips
and colds can begin to emerge. A concentrated source of vitamin C, lycopene and
ellagic acid, rosehips' antioxidant benefits can support us through winter. Prized
in traditional medicine for ailments such as osteoarthritis, they also assist collagen
production. You will need a muslin (cheesecloth) to strain the juice.

INGREDIENTS

~ 1.5kg (3lb 5oz/7½ cups) rosehips

~ 1.5 litres (52fl oz/6 cups) water

~ 5 cloves

~ 3–6 tbsp raw honey

MAKES
About 1 litre
(34fl oz/4 cups)

METHOD

Remove the stalks and wash the rosehips. Roughly chop or
blitz for a few seconds in a powerful blender or food processor.
You want the fruit to be smashed or broken for maximum
infusion. Tip into a large saucepan, add 1 litre (34fl oz/4 cups)
of the water and the cloves and bring to the boil, then reduce
to a gentle simmer for 20 minutes.

Line a sieve (fine mesh strainer) with muslin and stand
it over a large jug. Pour in the mixture and twist the muslin
to strain thoroughly. Tip the fruity pulp back into the
saucepan and cover with the remaining 500ml (17fl oz/
2 cups) of water. Bring to the boil, then turn the heat
off and leave to steep for 1 hour before repeating the
straining process. Pour into sterilised bottles or jars.

Storage: Keep in the refrigerator for up to 3 weeks.
Dose: Drink a shot neat or add to sparkling water as a
winter cordial as often as you like.
NOTE: Honey is not suitable for children under 1 year.

MAKES
About 200g
(7oz)

SCAR TREATMENT CREAM

I thought it would be important to include in this chapter the most literal and visceral of healing – to help reduce and smooth out the wounds of a scar. This cream works for older and newer scars as well as stretch marks, or any skin tissue that needs help to heal, making it a super-thoughtful present for a new mother or someone just out of hospital from surgery. The rosehip oil softens and brightens skin, while the shea and cocoa butters are nourishing and replenishing.

I N G R E D I E N T S ~ 100g (3½oz) shea butter ~ 50g (1¾oz) cocoa butter

~ 3 tbsp olive oil ~ 2 tbsp rosehip oil

M E T H O D Place all the ingredients in a large Kilner (Mason) jar, then stand the jar in a pan of boiling water until the ingredients have melted. Once melted, use a hand-held blender to whip the softened ingredients together to form a creamy substance. Pour or scrape into a 200g (7oz/scant ½ cup) jar, label and leave to cool. **Storage:** Keeps for up to 12 months. **Dose:** Apply daily.

COLD SORE PROTECTION LEMON LIP BALM

Prevention is always preferable to suffering the blight that cold sores can be, and this lip balm can be used regularly to keep them at bay. Lemon balm is active against the herpes virus so it should help both treat and prevent.

MAKES
About 1
tablespoon

I N G R E D I E N T S ~ 1 tsp beeswax pellets ~ 1 tsp cocoa butter ~ 10 drops of lemon balm essential oil ~ 5 drops of lemon essential oil

M E T H O D Melt the beeswax and cocoa butter in a small bowl over a pan of boiling water – or place it in a mug in the pan. Mix in the oils, pour into a small jar and leave to set, then seal and label.

Storage: Keeps for up to 4 months. **Dose:** Rub a little onto the lips regularly

TIP: Always label and date anything you store in a bottle. You may think you'll remember what it is, but you may not! Permanent markers work so well on glass and don't require sticky label removal.

LIVER TONIC

The organ that works so hard to process the toxins that live in and around us constantly can be over-burdened at night, particularly if we eat and drink late, and this combination can impact our sleep. There are still schools of thought that question the need for detoxing of any kind, but it makes clear and discernible sense to me that the clean-up apparatus would benefit immeasurably from its own scouring. Lemons are used in many natural cleaning products and also make an effective internal cleanser; their refreshing juice supports the liver's natural functioning. Combined with beetroot for potassium and antioxidants, and carrots for their liver-protecting retinoic acid.

INGREDIENTS

~ 1 lemon, peeled

~ 1 beetroot, topped, tailed and quartered

~ 1 carrot, peeled and roughly chopped

~ 5cm (2in) ginger root, peeled

METHOD

In a juicer, juice all the ingredients and drink immediately for optimal nutritional benefit, although you can make double the quantity and store the remainder.

Storage: Keep the remainder in a glass bottle in the refrigerator for up to a week.

Dose: Use daily as required.

MAKES
One serving

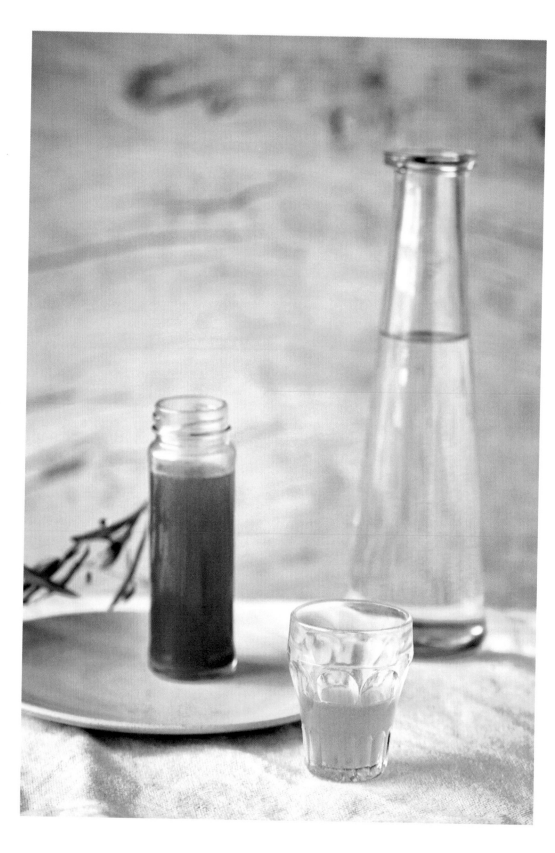

GUT-BOOSTING MORNING SHOT

This is a short drink to feed the bacteria in the gut and maximise the health of the environment where our microbiome lives. The studies linking gut health and immunity, as well as long-term health and chronic diseases, are becoming increasingly compelling, so a shot in the morning is a great insurance policy and particularly helpful if you're coming down with anything.

INGREDIENTS

~ 1 tbsp apple cider vinegar

~ ½ tsp raw honey

~ 100ml (3½fl oz/scant ½ cup) filtered water

METHOD

Pour the vinegar and honey into a glass, stirring the water through to mix, then drink at once. For greatest impact, drink on an empty stomach.

Storage: Make fresh as required.

Dose: Drink daily on an empty stomach.

NOTE: Honey is not suitable for children under 1 year.

MAKES
One drink

SAGE & ROSEMARY EARACHE STEAM

Many earaches will settle themselves, but steaming the airways
can ease congestion, relieve pressure and soothe all at once.
Do consult a doctor if the earache persists.

INGREDIENTS

~ 1 tbsp chopped sage leaves

~ 1 tbsp roughly chopped rosemary leaves

~ boiling water

METHOD

Put the herbs in a large basin or bowl and pour over boiling water to cover. Lean over the steaming basin with a towel draped over the back of your head, close your eyes and breathe deeply for 5–10 minutes to inhale the steam.

Storage: Make fresh as required.

Dose: Use twice a day as needed.

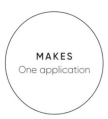

MAKES
One application

COLD & FLU SOOTHING CLOVE & CINNAMON TEA

This refreshing infusion is full of beneficial antioxidants. The warming properties of the herbs are helpful to relieve phlegm and mucus from the lungs while soothing sore throats. Cloves are strong on antiseptic and antivirals, and the cinnamon lends a gentle sweetness, but do add honey if you need more.

INGREDIENTS

~ 1 cinnamon stick

~ a few cloves

~ 500ml (17fl oz/2 cups) boiling water

~ raw honey, to taste (optional)

METHOD

Add the herbs to a large teapot and pour over the boiling water. Leave to infuse for 5 minutes. Pour into a teacup and sip, adding a teaspoon of honey to taste if you like.

Storage: Make fresh as required.

Dose: Sip a cup as often as you like.

NOTE: Honey is not suitable for children under 1 year.

MAKES
About 500ml
(17fl oz/2 cups)

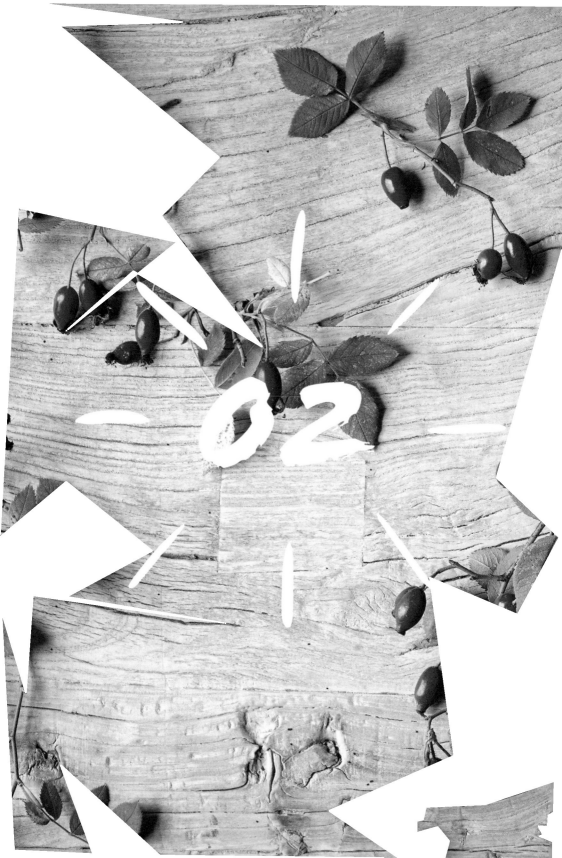

CALM

This chapter is all about natural downtime – bath soaks, hair masks, steam remedies and beyond – the best ways of keeping calm and staying natural. Often regarded as treats, activities like a soak in a bath, a time out with a face mask or just some reading or staring out of the window can make a world of a difference to our stress and cortisol levels, anxiety and general mood – which in turn has an impact on our ability to fight off disease and stay well.

Most of these recipes are aids to winding down and I have used them over the years when I just felt like a pick-me-up after a long day or when illness seemed to be on the horizon. Others I have discovered more recently, like the rose petal bath bombs that my daughter came up with – and we now have added pink fizz to bath time.

LAVENDER PILLOW SPRAY

The idea of spritzing your bed linen to welcome a better night's sleep is no longer novel, but the difference it makes and the joy of being able to tweak it to your own strength and taste is so pleasing – and saves you pennies, of course. A lovely present this one, in a pretty spray bottle with a ribbon and a handwritten label.

INGREDIENTS

~ 15 drops of lavender essential oil

~ 3 tbsp witch hazel (or vodka)

~ 3 tbsp filtered water

~ 1 tsp dried lavender flowers (optional)

METHOD

Drop the oils and witch hazel or alcohol into a 100ml (3½fl oz/scant 1¼ cup) spray bottle. Fill up with filtered water and shake. Add some dried lavender flowers for distilling and aesthetics, if you can.

Shake the bottle, then spritz pillows and/or bed linen 15 minutes before you go to sleep and dream sweet dreams.

Storage: Stays fresh for up to 6 months.

Dose: Spritz your pillow liberally every day before bedtime.

MAKES
About 100ml
(3½fl oz/scant
½ cup)

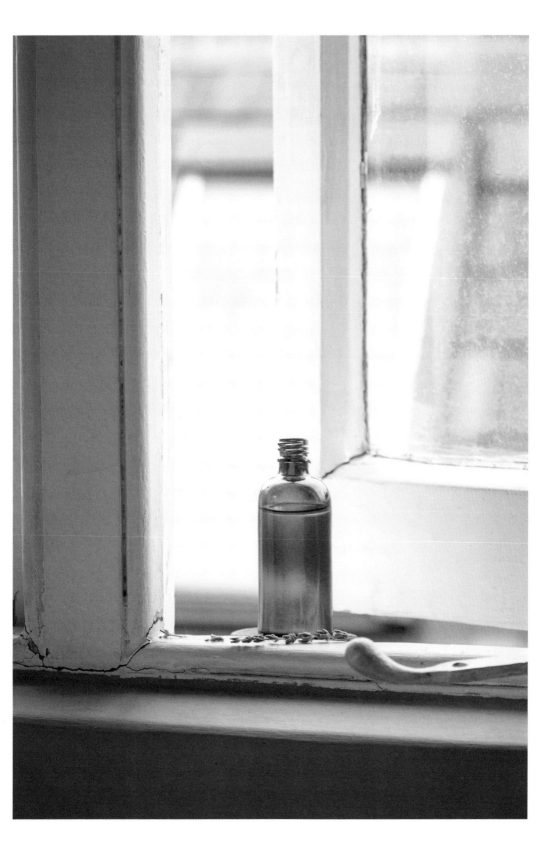

ROSEMARY & HIMALAYAN RECOVERY BATH SOAK

With the much-lauded Epsom and Himalayan salts to replenish minerals for your muscles, combined with mind-sharpening rosemary, add a large handful into a running bath, soaking for at least 10 minutes to nurture and revive.

INGREDIENTS

~ 200g (7oz/heaped 1½ cups) Himalayan salt

~ 200g (7oz/scant 1 cup) Epsom salts

~ 2 tsp fractionated coconut oil

~ 15 drops of rosemary essential oil

~ 1 tbsp fresh rosemary, roughly chopped (leave out if you prefer less bath rinsing)

METHOD

Combine the salts in a large bowl and add the oils and herbs. Mix together well and pour into a large jar. Label and seal.

Storage: Keeps for up to 6 months.

Dose: Use as often as you like.

TIP: Fractionated coconut oil remains liquid where standard coconut oil solidifies. It is readily available in health food stores.

MAKES
About 400g
(14oz/2½ cups)

ELECTROLYTE RESTORATION TONIC

After sick bugs or post-sport exertion, we need replenishment of the minerals that are vital to many key functions of the body, like sodium, calcium and potassium. I learnt this from a doctor in Switzerland years ago after a terrible sickness bug had left me nil by mouth for a couple of days. He seemed perplexed I didn't know this trick and scribbled down the ingredients. Simple to put together – and happily without all the E numbers from colours, flavours and preservatives of those on sale – it is the tonic my family all use now in place of sports drinks and after any illness to restore us to health.

INGREDIENTS

~ 600ml (20fl oz/2½ cups) water

~ 200ml (7fl oz/scant 1 cup) freshly squeezed orange juice

~ 100ml (3½fl oz/scant ½ cup) lemon juice

~ 1 tbsp raw honey

~ ½ tsp sea salt flakes or Himalayan salt

METHOD

Put all the ingredients into a 1 litre (34fl oz/4 cup) bottle and shake to mix, or blend together, then refrigerate for use as needed.

Storage: Make fresh as required and store in the refrigerator.

Dose: Drink the full bottle after exercise or sip it slowly over the course of 6 hours after sickness.

NOTE: Honey is not suitable for children under 1 year.

MAKES
About 1 litre
(34fl oz/4 cups)

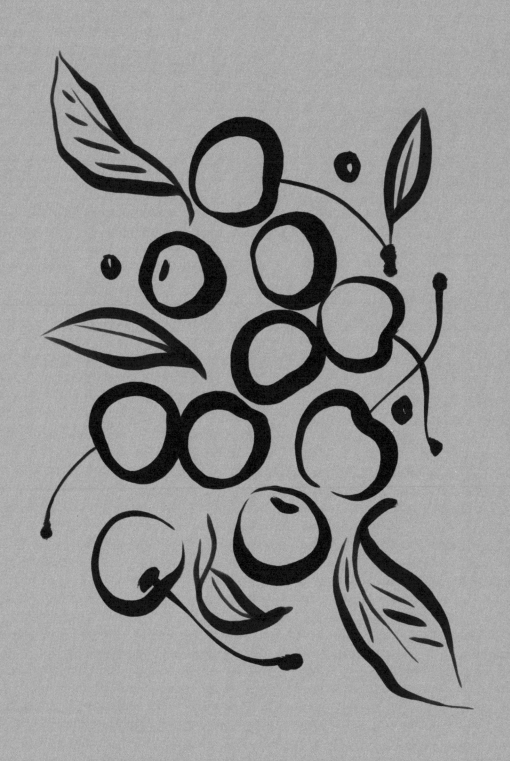

SPOTLIGHT ON
MONTMORENCY CHERRY

The Montmorency variety of cherry is most notable for its tartness and for providing relief from arthritis and gout. It is being highlighted here for being one of the only natural food sources of melatonin, a hormone that helps regulate sleep. Thought to be named after the French valley north of Paris where the noble family cultivated it in the 13th century, the bright red-fleshed, sour variety now makes up 95% of the American tart cherry industry.

A small trial in 2017* on insomniacs showed that, on average, they had 84 minutes more sleep a night than those who did not. Their blood tests showed elevated levels of tryptophan, an amino acid that is the precursor to melatonin, and decreased levels of inflammatory markers, which can disrupt sleep. As well as having a distinctive taste, the side effects of the tart cherry have so far only proved to be positive – as an effective muscle relief after exercise, and to help ease the effects of gout.

* Subjects in the trial by Louisiana University were given either a placebo drink or 230 ml (8 oz) Montmorency cherry juice 1–2 hours before bed

SLEEP TIGHT SMOOTHIE

Sleep can be so elusive as a parent but so crucial to stay sane and keep well. I came up with this after a particularly hideous clock-change week that left us devoid of rest in the evening or early mornings. It is a specially formulated smoothie, with a few natural ingredients picked for their combined calming and relaxing properties for body and mind, to encourage you to go to sleep faster and for longer. As well as the natural melatonin from the cherry concentrate, bananas are high in calming potassium. It's especially useful for any routine disruptions – before exams, after holidays, as well as the obvious ones like jet lag and clock changes when restless nights can send everyone wildly off track. This was put together to try to help reset your circadian rhythm whenever you need.

INGREDIENTS

~ 1 tbsp sour cherry concentrate

~ 1 banana

~ 250g (9oz/1 cup) plain yogurt

~ 1 tsp raw honey, to taste

METHOD

Put the cherry concentrate into a blender with the banana and yogurt, blend, then serve immediately with a straw.

Storage: Make fresh as required.

Dose: Drink a glass before you go to bed.

NOTE: Honey is not suitable for children under 1 year.

MAKES
About 300g
(10½oz/scant
1¼ cups)

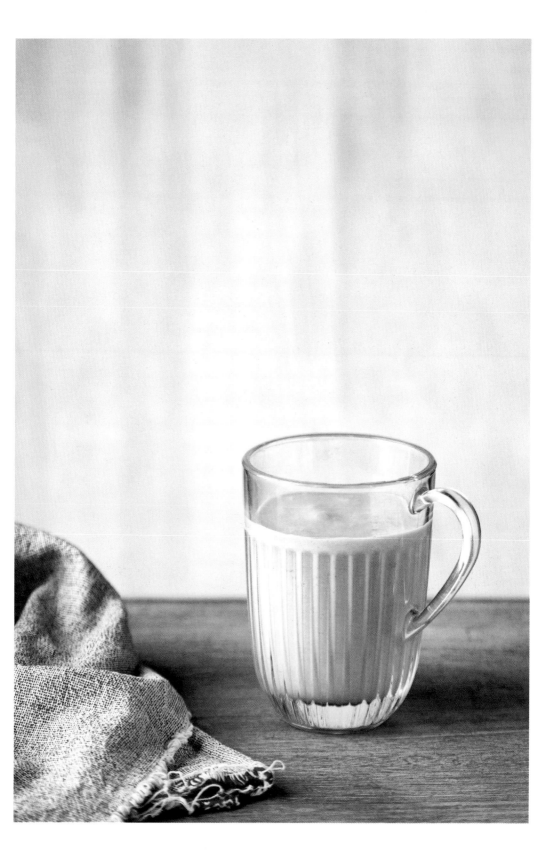

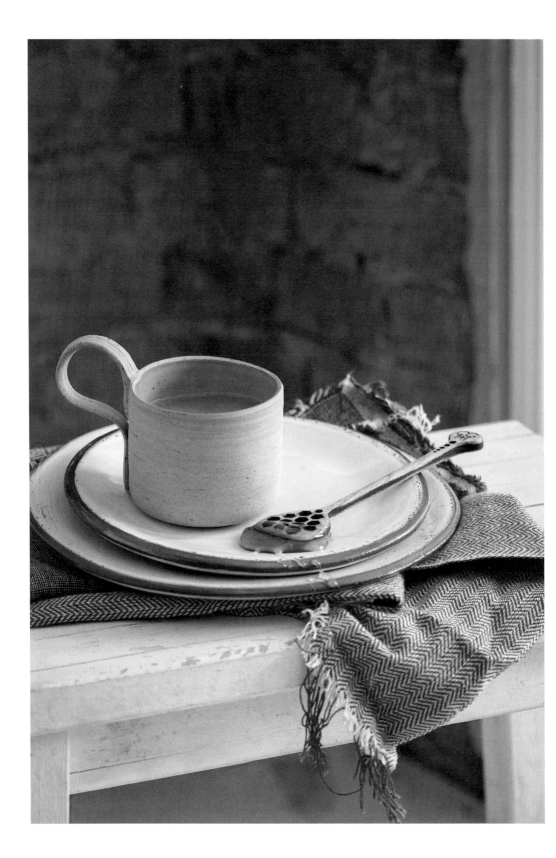

MUSHROOM BEDTIME COCOA

Cocoa has long been a soothing evening drink, and adding adaptogenic mushrooms means it can help with stress relief and hormone imbalance. I'm using reishi mushroom here for its sleep-promoting properties but you can also use alternatives: chaga, lion's mane or cordyceps mushroom powders all have a host of benefits and immune-supporting qualities. You can buy them online or in health food stores.

INGREDIENTS

~ 1 tsp reishi mushroom powder

~ 1 tbsp cocoa (unsweetened chocolate) powder

~ 200ml (7fl oz/scant 1 cup) milk of choice

~ 1 cinnamon stick

~ raw honey, to taste

METHOD

Mix the powders with the milk in a small saucepan. Add the cinnamon stick and whisk as you warm the mixture over a low heat for 5 minutes. Remove the cinnamon stick. Pour the milk into a mug and serve with a dash of honey to taste.

Storage: Make fresh as required.

Dose: Drink a mug before you go to bed.

NOTE: Honey is not suitable for children under 1 year.

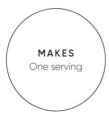

MAKES
One serving

DECONGESTANT NIGHT-TIME VAPOUR RUB

Clearing the airways for children at bedtime can make all the difference to recovery time from a cough or cold, and this simple eucalyptus rub can ease congestion when used on the chest. Over 75% of Australian vegetation is made up of this ancient tree, which was first used by the indigenous peoples, who chewed the roots and drank eucalyptus tea for fevers.
Adding about 10 drops of eucalyptus essential oil into a bowl of steaming water, leaning over it with a towel draped over the head and breathing deeply can be a very effective pre-bedtime steam inhalation, too.

INGREDIENTS

~ 1 tbsp shea butter

~ 2 tbsp beeswax pellets

~ 3 tbsp coconut oil

~ 10 drops of eucalyptus essential oil

~ 5 drops of lemon essential oil

METHOD

Using a heatproof bowl over a saucepan of boiling water, melt the shea butter, beeswax and coconut oil. Add the oils and stir together. Pour into jars and leave to cool until solidified, then seal and label.

Storage: Stays fresh for up to 12 months.

Dose: Rub about a teaspoonful of the balm – depending on the size of the area! – onto the chest and back before bedtime when blocked up, stuffy or coldy. Also effective on the soles of the feet.

MAKES
About 100ml
(3½fl oz/scant
½ cup)

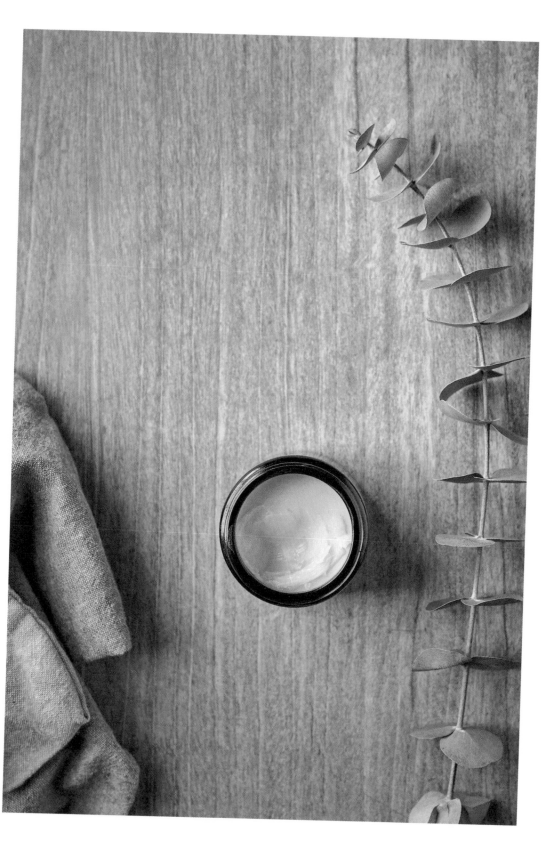

HANGOVER HELPER

I'm not sure science would argue that anything can undo the work of a hangover, but this blood-sugar-stabilising tonic should ease heads and stomachs and hopefully prevent too many cravings. The microbiome is impacted by alcohol, so this gut bacteria replenishment should also help right that imbalance, with the minerals that are often missing after a big night – potassium, sodium and magnesium – included.

INGREDIENTS ~ 1 tbsp apple cider vinegar ~ pinch of sea salt flakes

~ 1 tsp raw honey ~ 200ml (7fl oz/scant 1 cup) water

METHOD Mix all the ingredients together and drink immediately.

Storage: Make fresh as required. Dose: Use as often as needed.

MAKES
One serving

SUNBURN RESPITE TEA WRAP

The polyphenols – specifically the tannic acid and theobromine – found in tea can be soothing and healing to sun-damaged skin, and if you are far from a shop and need to use the kitchen cupboard, this is an uncomplicated formula to soothe and ease discomfort.

INGREDIENTS ~ 5 green or black tea bags ~ 300ml (10½floz/scant 1¼ cups) boiling water

METHOD Steep the tea bags in the boiling water for 10 minutes, then remove. Saturate a clean tea towel or kitchen paper in the tea, then place in the refrigerator to cool. Gently place the material on the affected skin as needed, patting to apply, and leave for 10 minutes.

Storage: Make fresh as required. Dose: Apply as needed.

MAKES
One
application

FROZEN YOGURT EYE BAG RELIEF

Puffy, dark circles are an immediate sign that we need to take more care of ourselves and usually the first thing to warrant others telling us how tired we look. This very straightforward eye mask works so well in reducing puffiness as well as dark bags, with its lactic acid to brighten and turmeric to reduce inflammation. As a Sunday night ritual or before an event I want to look sprightly for, this instantly makes me feel brighter and sparklier. That makes it great to boost your general wellbeing, too.

INGREDIENTS ~ 3 tbsp plain yogurt ~ 1 tsp ground turmeric

METHOD Mix the ingredients until well combined. You can use it immediately, spreading it evenly under your eyes and relaxing for 10–15 minutes before washing it off.

Alternatively, you can freeze it for a harder hit. Using a sheet of greaseproof (waxed) paper, hold it up to your eyes and draw a u-shaped under-eye outline on the paper from your lower lid to your cheekbones. Spread the yogurt mixture within the lines and freeze for 1 hour. Peel the paper backing off when needed and press the frozen mask onto your under eye area. Relax for 10–15 minutes, then wash off.

Storage: Make as required or freeze a larger quantity for up to a month.

Dose: Once a week or as required.

TIP: You can make a larger quantity of the eye masks – say, 6 treatments – and leave them in the freezer so they are ready whenever you want them.

MAKES
One
treatment

ARNICA & GINGER PAIN RELIEF SALVE

Bruises, muscle aches, joint stiffness, over-exercising – any of these pains can be relieved with this magical mixture. Arnica has been a saviour of mine with young children and I've seen how effective it is on bumps and bruises. This salve can be rubbed in topically for anything causing pain but do not use on broken skin.

INGREDIENTS

~ 2 tbsp beeswax pellets

~ 1 tbsp shea butter

~ 80ml (2½fl oz/⅓ cup) arnica oil

~ 1 tsp ginger essential oil

METHOD

Using a heatproof bowl over a saucepan of boiling water, melt the beeswax and shea butter, stirring gently. Add the oils and combine well. Pour into 30ml (2 tbsp) brown glass, lidded jars and leave to cool. When hardened, seal and label.

Storage: Keep in a cool, dark place for up to 3 months.

Dose: Rub on unbroken skin as required.

TIP: You can infuse your own arnica oil with the arnica flower.

MAKES
About 120ml
(4fl oz/scant
½ cup)

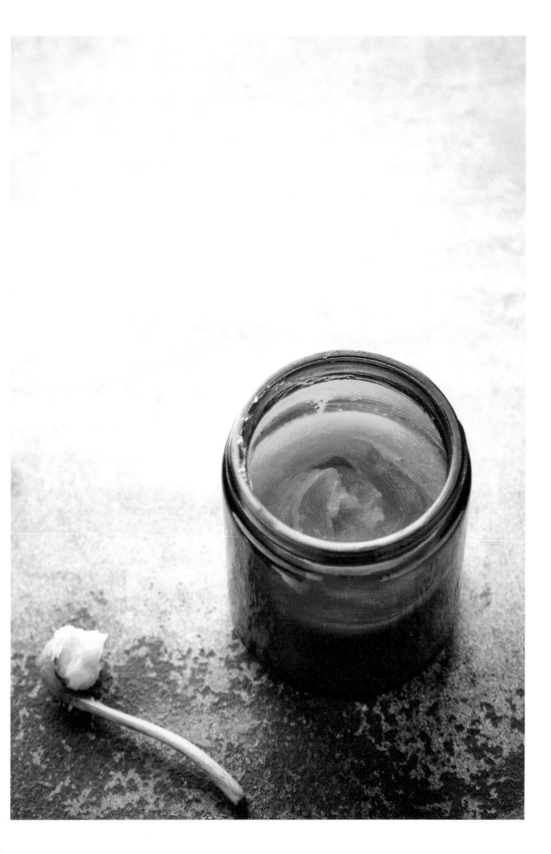

REMEDIES FOR DOGS

In much the same way that feeding my own children focused my mind on reading up on the received wisdom and challenging many of the often substandard norms, when we got our first family puppy, Bobby, I started reading labels and querying some of the things that were being proffered by marketing companies, big pharma and the hugely profitable pet food industry.

Diet is the obvious starting point for all health, so do look at how you are feeding your dog. Healthy, well-nourished pets are less likely to suffer from most ailments, including fleas, joint issues and diarrhoea.

Our pets are treasured members of the family and they come with no guidance, so the information flung at us is often latched on to with desperation and relief as an answer to an immediate problem. From fleas to sore paws, runny tummies and licked wounds, there are ways to help that are simple, effective, money-saving and even fun.

NOTE: I am not a dog expert or trained veterinarian, so do please seek help from your vet or trusted dog expert. My go-to dog behaviourist, Louise Glazebrook, is an endless resource for how to do best by your pup. Her book, *The Book Your Dog Wishes You Would Read*, is a godsend. She also holds puppy classes, takes individual clients and even makes her own dog treats and behaviour boxes. Visit **www.darlingdogcompany.co.uk**

CHARCOAL RICE DOG SICKNESS TREATMENT

While we know exactly what goes in their dog bowl at meal times, we have less idea about what they hoover up elsewhere or if any bugs are going round. Dogs getting bad tummies may be reasonably common but can be worrying, particularly when they are new to us or young. Some breeds are also more sensitive in the stomach so it's always a relief to have something you know can help.

INGREDIENTS ~ 1–3 activated charcoal capsules ~100–300g (3½–10oz/⅔–1⅔ cups) plain boiled rice ~ 2–3 tbsp chicken stock (or use Dog Joint & Digestion Bone Broth Jelly, page 67)

METHOD Combine all three ingredients and feed to your dog after an episode of diarrhoea or sickness. **Storage:** Make fresh as required. **Dose:** Serve instead of their usual food after an episode of sickness or diarrhoea. **NB:** If there is blood in their poo, they are lethargic or not eating, please seek veterinarian help if needed or if the problem persists.

MAKES
One
serving

ROUGH PAW BALM

Wet, cold winter months can cause the sensitive paw pads to roughen up. Smooth this balm over their paws daily while you both enjoy stroking them. And if they lick it straight off, there are only good things going in.

INGREDIENTS ~ 2 tbsp coconut oil ~ 1 tbsp shea butter ~ 1 tbsp beeswax pellets ~ 1 tsp olive oil

METHOD Place all the ingredients into a large mug. Pour boiling water into a small saucepan and sit the mug in it until the contents have melted. Use a hand-held blender to blend together, then pour into a jar and allow to set, which could take up to 6 hours. Seal and label.

Storage: Keeps for up to 6 months. **Dose:** Rub a teaspoonful on the paws daily.

MAKES
About 60ml
(4 tbsp)

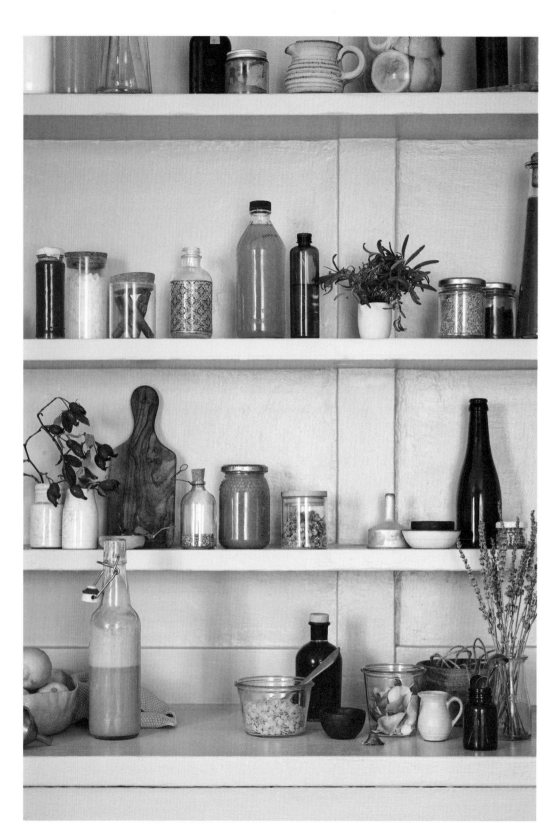

APPLE VINEGAR FLEA SPRAY

The incessant itching from flea bites can often lead to nasty wounds if an animal tries to scratch or gnaw at the offending bites to get some relief from the irritation. This is an easily made spray that provides a good protection against fleas. As well as everyday prevention, the inhospitable acidic environment it creates on the fur makes fleas less likely to be interested in staying around.

INGREDIENTS

~ 300ml (10½fl oz/scant 1¼ cups) water

~ 1 tbsp chopped rosemary leaves

~ 3 tbsp apple cider vinegar

~ juice of ½ lemon

~ 1 tsp sea salt flakes

METHOD

Bring the water to the boil in a small saucepan, add the rosemary, reduce the heat and simmer for 15 minutes; the smell will be deliciously fragrant. Remove from the heat and leave to cool. Combine the water with the remaining ingredients in a spray bottle and shake to combine.

Storage: Stays fresh for up to 3 months.

Dose: Spray onto the skin once every 2–3 days, brushing through the fur and on the belly to keep fleas away.

MAKES
About 350ml
(12¼fl oz/1½ cups)

WOUND & ITCH RELIEF

Foods, environment, heat and cleaning products can all cause a reaction in
dogs in the same way it can with us, but as they can't tell us, it is our job to
notice any changes to their coats, flaky skin: itching and so on. First of all,
investigate why you think your dog has any itching or flaky skin, and discuss
the best plan for treating that long term. Working out the food or irritant
could involve an elimination diet. If you dog suffers a wound, it will tend to
lick it, and although this is often healing, sometimes it can lead to a wound
remaining open and wet, in which case it can become worse day by day –
and they end up being given cones to wear to prevent this.

INGREDIENTS

~ 1 tsp sea salt flakes

~ 2 tbsp cooled boiled water

~ 1 tbsp coconut oil

MAKES
Any quantity

METHOD

To encourage a wound to heal, make a saline solution
with the salt and water and use it to gently wash the area
before applying coconut oil. The antibacterial properties
will support healing.

To deal with itching skin, gently rub a little coconut
oil into any dry, flaky patches to relieve the itching.

Storage: Make fresh as required.

Dose: Apply to the skin as needed.

TIP: You can also add a spoonful of coconut oil to
their food to help from within.

FRESH BREATH TREATS

Keeping our dogs' teeth healthy and strong is important in keeping them pain free as well as in good health, eating what they are accustomed to and chewing on things they love. Poor dental health can also mean bad breath, so combatting both here is the aim. These treats keep teeth clean and breath fresh.

INGREDIENTS ~ 4 tbsp coconut oil ~ 1 tbsp chopped parsley ~ ½ tsp ground turmeric

METHOD Melt the coconut oil and combine with the other ingredients. Pour into small ice-cube trays or moulds and refrigerate until set, which will take up to an hour.

Storage: Keeps in the refrigerator for a few days. **Dose:** Feed one tablespoon-sized cube a day to your dog.

MAKES
About 10–15
biscuits,
depending
on size

PEANUT BUTTER TREATS

Baking your own dog chews may seem an extra mile to go when there are so many out there, plenty of which are good quality. But I loved putting this together with some of my youngest son's favourite things. It seemed a delicious treat for a perfect puppy.

INGREDIENTS ~ 200g (7oz/1¾ cups) coconut flour ~ 3 tbsp milled linseed (flaxseed) ~ ½ tsp ground cinnamon ~ 2 bananas ~ 200g (7oz/¾ cup) peanut butter ~3 eggs ~ 1 tbsp olive oil ~ water

METHOD Heat the oven to 160°C (320°F/gas 3) and line a baking sheet with baking parchment. Combine the dry ingredients in a large bowl. Mash the bananas well, then mix in the eggs, peanut butter and olive oil. Add the wet mixture gradually into the dry, stirring gently, then pour in a little water at a time until you have a mixture that holds together but is not runny. Shape the mixture into dog bones (or whatever you fancy) or gently roll it out and use a cookie cutter. Bake for 20–25 minutes, then leave to cool on a wire rack.

Storage: Keep in an airtight container. **Dose:** Serve as a treat, once a day.

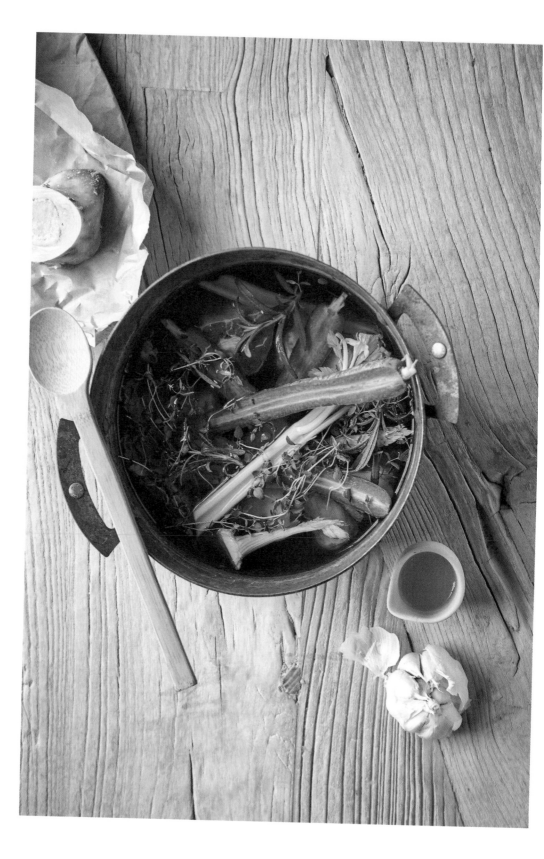

DOG JOINT & DIGESTION BONE BROTH JELLY

Joint health is critical to keeping dogs active and happy into old age, and boiling up your own tasty broth provides critical joint-strengthening nutrients – glucosamine and glycine – and amino acids to help collagen production. It is also a great gut-soothing recipe for dogs who have had a bad tummy. I like storing this in large ice-cube moulds, then turning one out and serving at room temperature. The texture should be jelly-like, so if it is runny the first time you make it, increase the cooking time or add less water during the simmering stage.

INGREDIENTS

~ 1.3kg (3lb) beef bones (use marrow bones and a joint bone, too, if you can)

~ 2 tbsp apple cider vinegar

~ 2 celery stalks, roughly chopped

~ 2 carrots, peeled and roughly chopped

~ 1 sprig of rosemary

~ 1 sprig of thyme

~ 2 garlic cloves, peeled

~ water

MAKES
About 3 litres
(105fl oz/12 cups)

METHOD

Place the bones in a large saucepan (or slow cooker). Tuck the other ingredients in between the bones and pour in enough water to reach 2.5cm (1in) over the bones. Bring to the boil, then reduce the heat, cover and simmer gently for 7–12 hours, checking the water level and topping up with boiling water as needed.

Remove and discard the bones – don't be tempted to feed them to your dog, as once boiled they can splinter and be very dangerous.

You can serve ladles of this fresh and warm, or spoon over dry kibbles. Leave to cool, then remove any fat that solidifies on the surface. Pour into giant ice-cube moulds (or you could use lolly moulds) and freeze, then serve 2–3 tablespoons with their food, or alone if needing a stomach soothe or for digestive problems.

Storage: Freeze for up to 3 months.

Dose: 2–3 tablespoons a day with food or on its own.

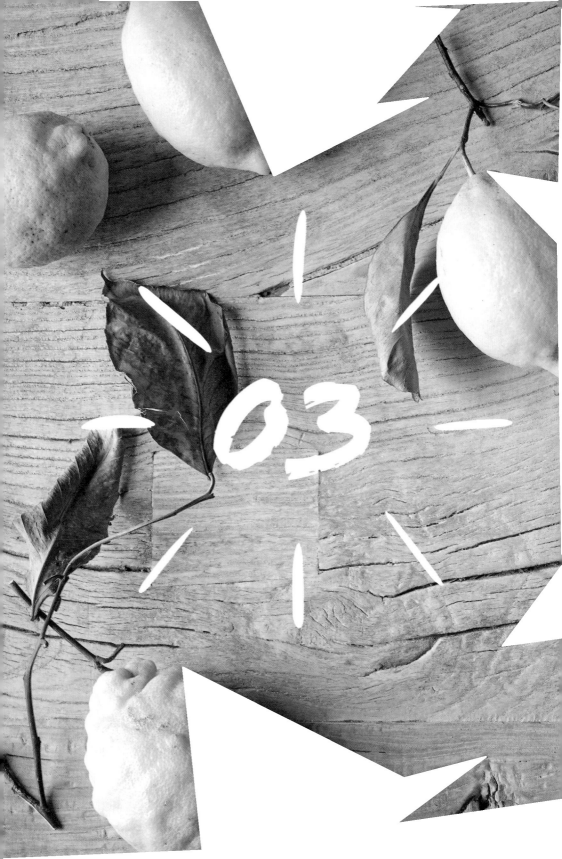

PAMPER

The labels on food and their provenance were certainly the gateway for me scrutinising the products my family and I were using in the bathroom every day. As new-borns, I used olive oil on my children's skin to start with, and moving from the purity of that single, gloriously edible ingredient to the pungent pots of products on sale felt wrong. I began buying brands that were transparent and spartan with their ingredients, using fewer and usually natural elements that I could recognise. Then I realised it wasn't so hard to make bath soaks or balms.

As our largest organ, our skin is an incredibly efficient membrane, both absorbing elements from the outside and excreting those we no longer need. The beauty industry has recently come under scrutiny for using ingredients now deemed unsafe in many of our everyday creams and lotions. But labelling things 'chemical' and therefore bad, or 'natural' and therefore good, is far too reductive an approach. We have to work out our own personal preferences and thresholds.

With the combination of confidence as I put them together and satisfaction in their effectiveness, I wanted to share these beautiful bathroom creations with you.

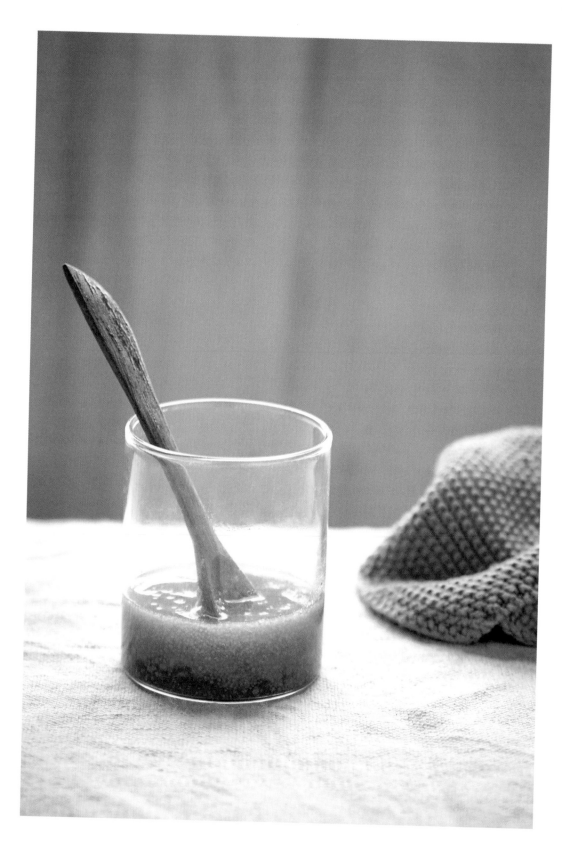

TIRED FACE HONEY MASK

Evenings in with boxsets and slippers can be upgraded with a bit of skin love. Face masks you put together yourself can be way cheaper and easier than shop-bought versions – plus you know you can lick your fingers afterwards. This failsafe honey mask leaves you with a dewy glow and more of the good bugs on your skin surface. And it has just one magic ingredient.

INGREDIENTS

~ 3 tbsp raw honey

~ warm water as needed

METHOD

Spread the honey carefully over your face, warming it gently in a pan if you need to make it more spreadable. Leave for 10–20 minutes. Rinse off with a hot cloth.

Storage: Make fresh as required.

Dose: Use once a week or as you like.

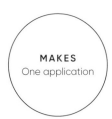

MAKES
One application

GLOSSY LOCKS SODA SCALP SCRUB

The delicate skin on our scalp needs to be in good health to ensure the hair follicles are provided with nourishment for strong, healthy, glossy hair. This is the simplest of scrubs, using bicarbonate of soda to reset the pH of your scalp and help resolve 'build-up' (beauty speak for all the sticky stuff in the products staying on the surface) and irritation, leaving silky, luscious locks. The coconut oil is a nourishing addition to prevent the bicarbonate from drying the scalp.

INGREDIENTS

~ 2 tbsp bicarbonate of soda (baking soda)

~ 1 tbsp coconut oil

~ water as needed

METHOD

Mix the coconut oil into the powder, then add a few drops of water at a time to create a paste.

Comb the hair into a parting and apply to the scalp, rubbing in well. Leave on for 10 minutes, then apply shampoo directly to the mixture before rinsing.

Storage: Make fresh as required.

Dose: Use once or twice a month.

MAKES
One application

FROZEN CHAMOMILE & CUCUMBER EYE SOOTHER

Sometimes we just want our tired, puffy, stinging eyes to feel some respite from life, and this lovely icy treatment is a glorious release and an instant relaxer. Chamomile is soothing and calming to the skin and cucumber reduces inflammation. Any tough days can be eased quickly with this treat.

INGREDIENTS

~ 3 chamomile tea bags (or 3 tsp dried chamomile flowers)

~ 300ml (10½fl oz/scant 1¼ cups) boiling water

~ ½ cucumber, chopped and blended

MAKES
About 12 ice cubes, depending on size of tray

METHOD

Make a strong mug of chamomile tea using the tea bags, or herbs, and boiling water, then leave to brew for 10 minutes.

Remove the bags and leave the tea to cool. Mix in the cucumber purée. Using a large ice-cube tray, pour the tea into the bottom of each section, but only fill up to about 2.5cm (1in).

Freeze for 2–3 hours until hardened, then pop them out and reserve in a labelled bag in the freezer.

To use, lie back and place a damp muslin (cheesecloth) over your whole face, then put a single piece over each of your eye sockets. Hold to your eyes as they melt and the liquid cools through the cloth and depuffs your eye area.

Storage: Freeze for up to 6 months.

Dose: Use as required.

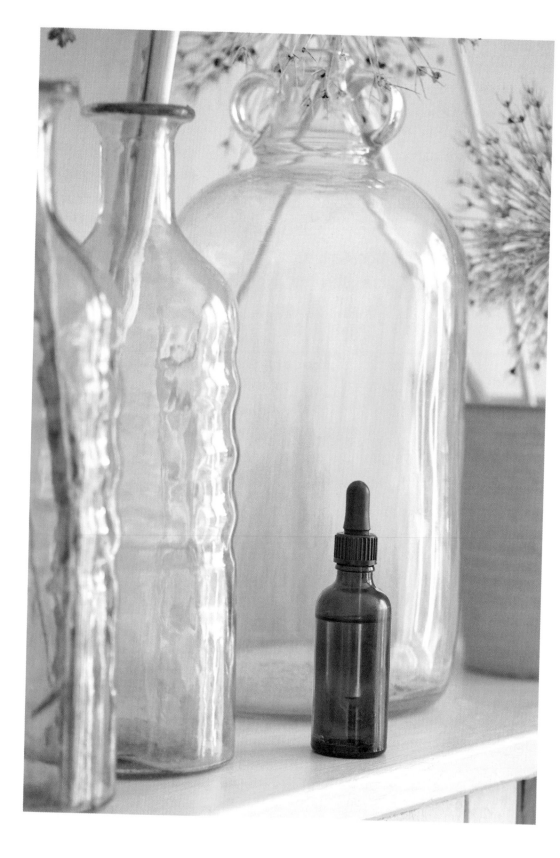

ORANGE & ALMOND OIL
HAND & NAIL TREATMENT

As a cook I am always using my hands – chopping, mixing, washing. They both work hard and are often on display so frequently need some extra care. I keep a small dropper bottle in my handbag to deal with dry, rough hands. I often suffer from hard patches down the edges of the nails, so softening them and the nail bed with this oil helps promote fitter, stronger nails and hands you'll want to show off.

INGREDIENTS

~ 2 tsp almond oil

~ 10 drops of orange essential oil

METHOD

Combine the oils in a small bowl or mug, then use a funnel to pour into a 15ml (1 tbsp) dropper bottle. Apply a few drops to the nail beds, cuticles and fingers, massage in, then leave to absorb.

Storage: Keeps for up to 6 months.

Dose: Apply as and when needed.

MAKES
About
1 tablespoon

TIGHTEN, TONE AND DE-PUFF ICE FACIAL

Cryotherapy, Wim Hoff's method and cold-water swimming have been climbing in popularity for the overall benefits they boast. British supermodel Kate Moss was onto this face-saver decades ago. After late nights partying, or no sleep at all, Kate purportedly used to ask for ice and a bowl on arrival at a photo shoot, as an instantaneous method to erase the evidence of the night before on her skin. An easy at-home facial treat, it works by reducing the puffiness straight away by constricting the capillaries in our face, reducing redness, tightening skin and boosting the lymph system. After the constriction, our skin is flooded with nutrients and oxygenated blood, giving us a dewy glow.

INGREDIENTS

~ 1 tray of large ice cubes

~ water

~ 1 tbsp apple cider vinegar (optional)

METHOD

Pop out the ice cubes into a large bowl, then add water until the bowl is three-quarters full. Add a splash of apple cider vinegar, if you wish. Tie your hair back or wear a headband, take a breath in and, closing your eyes, plunge your whole face under the water for 20–30 seconds at a time. Repeat a few times.

Storage: Keep a tray of ice cubes in the freezer for when you need them.

Dose: Use daily or whenever you need a depuff or de-stress session.

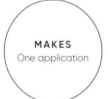

MAKES
One application

ROSEMARY & CHAMOMILE FACIAL STEAM

The most luxurious part of any facial for me, the steam alone freshens up tired, dull skin, opening up the pores to deep cleanse and hydrate. It also enables better absorption of products afterwards. Not only affecting the skin, this is also a mood-mellowing combination of chamomile, which is brightening, too, and antioxidant-rich rosemary. The increased blood flow during the steaming process promotes collagen and elastin production, all helping with the firm, dewy, youthful skin we're all after.

INGREDIENTS

~ 2 tsp chopped rosemary leaves

~ 2 tbsp herbs from chamomile teabags (or dried flowers)

~ 500ml (17fl oz/2 cups) boiling water

MAKES
One application

METHOD

Firstly, wash your face and tie back your hair, if needed. Place the herbs in a large bowl, pour over the just-boiled water, stir gently, and leave for a few minutes to cool slightly.

Sitting in a comfortable chair, place your head over the bowl, with a towel over your head to keep the steam in. Breathe deeply and relax for 5–10 minutes as the steam works on the skin. Pat dry, then splash your face with cold water to close the pores.

Storage: Make fresh as required.

Dose: Steam should only be used once or twice a week.

TIP: Alternatively, spritz with my Jasmine Morning Face Mist (page 88).

ROSE PETAL BATH BOMB

Please don't be put off if you think this is outside your skill set. I never would have billed myself as a pink fizz bath bomb crafter, but it was my daughter's idea, so we gave it a whirl and they've been a huge hit since. The children love patting these together and the effervescent finale is glorious. They are easy to assemble, a bit like pushing a snowball together, and they are so cheap to make, too. With only lovely things in them to go on your skin, you can switch up the added ingredients for your own flavours, colours, herbs or other flowers. And what a lovely present they make.

INGREDIENTS

~ 225g (8oz/1 cup) bicarbonate of soda (baking soda)

~ 125g (4½oz/½ cup) citric acid

~ 115g (4oz/½ cup) Epsom salts (or pink Himalayan salt to make them even pinker!)

~ 2 tsp strawberry powder

~ 2 tsp dried rose petals

~ 2 tbsp of rose or ylang ylang essential oil

~ 3 tsp almond oil (or use sunflower oil)

~ spray bottle with 2–6 tsp water

METHOD

Mix the dry powders and rose petals together in a large mixing bowl, and mix the oils in a small jug. Drip the oils slowly into the powder, drawing them together until the mixture packs together. Form into round balls, spritzing with the water as you go to keep them holding together.

Pack them into muffin tins, poached egg moulds or any spherical moulds and leave to dry out and harden overnight or for 24 hours.

Storage: Best made fresh but will keep for a few days.

Dose: Throw them in your bath and watch the wild pink fizz!

MAKES
About 12 bath bombs

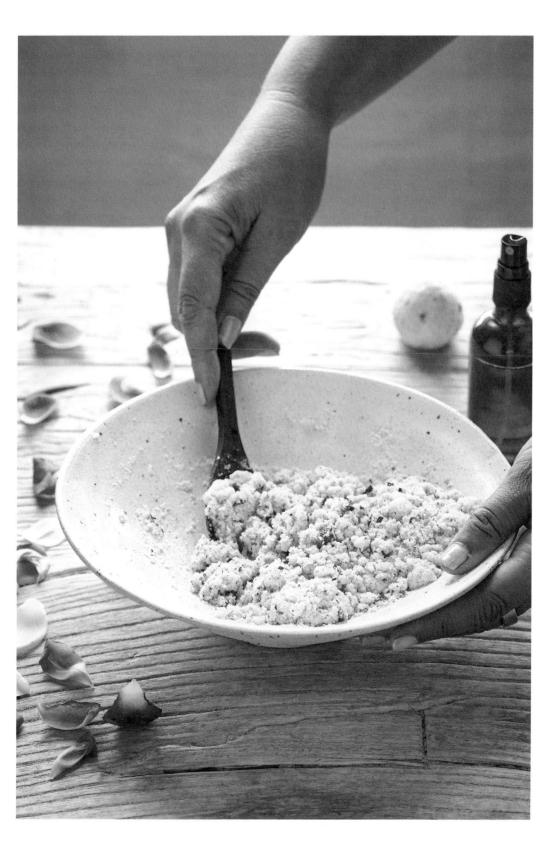

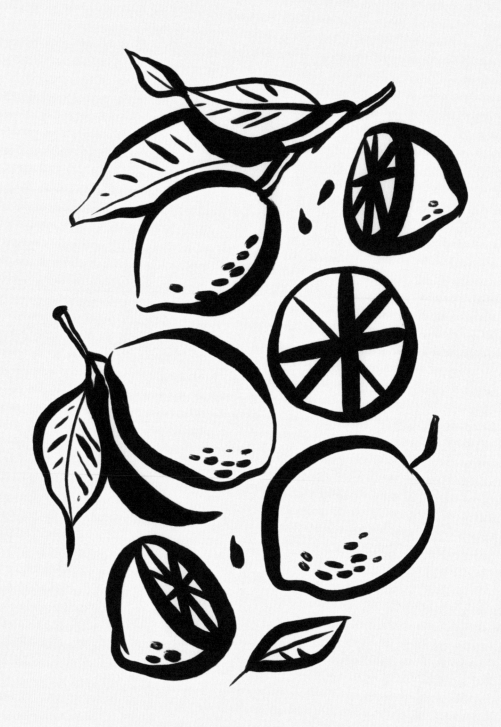

SPOTLIGHT ON
LEMON

The evergreen citron tree (*citrus medica*), from which came its relative the lemon (*citrus limon*), has been around for about 8 million years, with its astringent fruit having a multitude of uses, from culinary to medicinal, but also as an ingredient for preservation, beauty and cleaning purposes. The lemon's chemical make-up, with a high concentration of citric acid and ascorbic acid, means a low pH and that is at the core of most of the applications. One lemon contains 50mg of ascorbic acid (known more commonly as vitamin C), providing over half the daily requirement of this essential vitamin.

Used as a gastro remedy and antiseptic for the Ancient Egyptians, it was discovered to help prevent scurvy by a naval physician in 15th century. The acidic properties of the juice meant that as well as antibacterial uses it was used to make invisible ink, preserve food and polish furniture as well as embalm bodies. The zest provides an essential oil that brightens in skincare and freshens and uplifts as a scent. One of my most-used, multi-purpose ingredients, I often pack a single lemon in my suitcase to ensure I get fresh lemon squeezed into my first drink of the day.

TIP: Bringing the fruit up to room temperature means lemons will yield more juice, but storing them in water, in the fridge, will keep them fresh for up to 7 days.

KIDS' BEDTIME LEMON BATH SALTS

A heady, sleep-inducing bath of relaxation! As routine and bath time are ear-marked by all the experts as excellent tee-ups for a good night, I thought I'd supercharge the bath routine by adding minerals to it that help with muscle relaxing and de-stressing. The best part of this bath is that our systems – especially the kids' – can often be low on magnesium, a crucial nutrient, so this is nutrition while you bathe. It is a lovely, calming bath soak for adults, too – the relaxing magnesium can also help with back pain, headaches and relieving tension.

INGREDIENTS

~ 400g (14oz/heaped 1¾ cups) Epsom salts

~ 2 tbsp magnesium flakes

~ 10 drops of lemon essential oil

MAKES
About 450g
(1lb/2 cups)

METHOD

Combine all the ingredients in a large jar and shake well to mix.

Storage: Keep the jar in a cool, dry place for up to 3 months.

Dose: Add 2 handfuls to your bath under running water and bathe for at least 10 minutes to absorb the minerals. Double the dose if you are having trouble sleeping.

TIP: Epsom salts are rich in magnesium, so do use them alone if you don't have any magnesium flakes.

ROSEHIP BODY BALM

This is a creamy, rich body balm for beautifully bright skin. The high concentration of vitamin C in rosehips, as well as their skin-regenerating properties, means it nourishes, brightens and increases collagen production and is particularly good for healing on scars and pigmentation.

INGREDIENTS

~ 2 tbsp coconut oil

~ 1 tbsp beeswax pellets

~ 2 tbsp almond oil

~ 2 tbsp rosehip seed essential oil

~ 10 drops of geranium essential oil

METHOD

Warm the coconut oil with the beeswax and almond oil in a heatproof bowl sitting over a small saucepan of boiling water. Once melted and combined, remove from the heat and add the rosehip oil and geranium oil. Pour into a dark glass jar and leave to set. Label and screw on the lid.

Storage: Keeps in the jar in the refrigerator for up to 3 months.

Dose: Rub a small amount gently into the affected area every day.

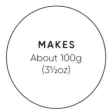

MAKES
About 100g
(3½oz)

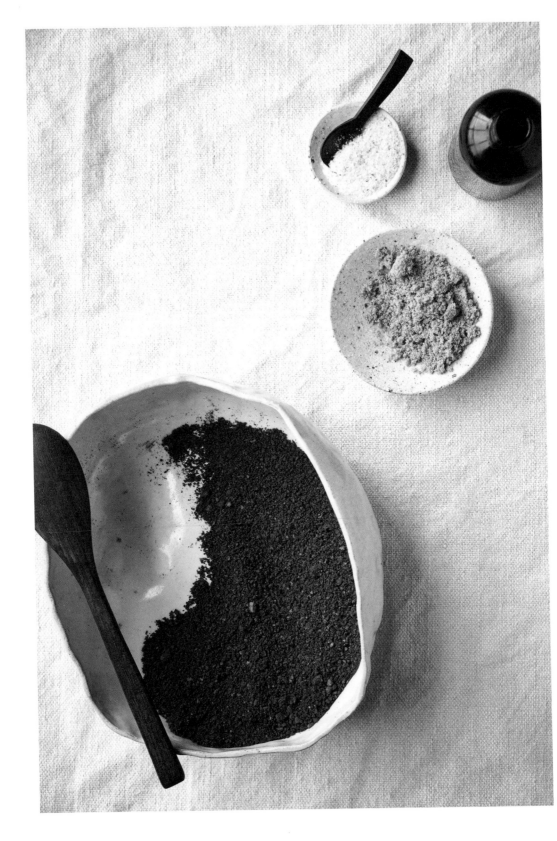

INVIGORATING COFFEE BODY SCRUB

Coffee famously has a host of stimulating and energising effects. And using up spent grinds, alongside coconut oil for a moisture boost, gives you a really gentle scrub that exfoliates the dead skin from the surface and encourages epidermal cell regeneration and thus softer, smoother, firmer skin. Caffeine is also said to be hard on cellulite due to the potent antioxidants it contains. Either way, it feels amazing and smells a little like an espresso martini, which helps!

INGREDIENTS

~ 90g (3¼oz/1 cup) coffee grinds

~ 2 tbsp Himalayan salt

~ 2 tbsp brown sugar

~ 120ml (4fl oz/½ cup) fractionated coconut oil (or melt regular coconut oil)

METHOD

Mix together the coffee, salt and sugar in a small bowl, then add the coconut oil and stir together with a wooden spoon. Store in a glass jar.

Storage: Store in the fridge for up to 3 months.
Dose: Either before or just after a bath, rub 1–2 tablespoons of the scrub from the legs upwards in a circular motion, always moving towards the heart. Rinse well with warm water.

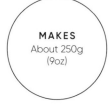

MAKES
About 250g
(9oz)

'KISS ME' BROWN SUGAR LIP SCRUB

Adorably easy and delicious to make, this will leave your lips soft, smooth
and sweet. The perfect party present to give in mini jars or leave as place settings
at a dinner party, whether or not you suffer from dry lips, you will be making
this on repeat and loving the kiss-ability it brings.

INGREDIENTS ~ 3 tbsp soft brown sugar (such as muscovado) ~ 2 tbsp olive oil
~ 2–3 drops of vanilla extract

METHOD Combine all the ingredients in a small bowl and break up any clumps while mixing the
oils into the sugar. Scoop into small jars. To use, dab onto lips and rub gently, using a soft cloth,
for 2–3 minutes. Rinse off, then apply lip balm.

Storage: Keeps in tightly sealed jar for up to 2 months. **Dose:** Use once a week or as required.

MAKES
About
80g (3oz)

COOLING ORANGE & MINT FOOT SOAK

This aromatic soak stimulates circulation, and calms and refreshes tired feet. The soothing effects of the aromatic orange and bay also alleviate aches and pains.

I N G R E D I E N T S ~ 15g (½oz/½ cup) mint leaves ~ 3 bay leaves ~ zest of 1 orange ~ boiling water ~ 10 drops of peppermint essential oil

M E T H O D Place the mint leaves, bay leaves and orange zest into a muslin (cheesecloth) bag and place in a large bowl. Pour over enough boiling water to cover, then leave to infuse for 5 minutes. If it is still too hot, add a little cold water until the temperature is comfortably warm for you, then add the peppermint oil and soak your feet for 10–20 minutes.

Storage: Make fresh as required. **Dose:** Use as required.

MAKES
One
application

SANDALWOOD ELBOW & KNEE SOFTENING BALM

A creamy, rich body balm, with skin-softening coconut oil whipped into moisturising almond oil to nourish and nurture the tough, rough patches on elbows and knees.

I N G R E D I E N T S ~ 3 tbsp coconut oil ~ 2 tbsp almond oil ~ 1 tbsp beeswax pellets ~ 2 tbsp sandalwood essential oil

M E T H O D Place the oils and beeswax into a large jar in a pan of boiling water until melted and combined. Carefully remove the jar from the pan and leave to cool for 10 minutes. Add the sandalwood oil and mix well. Pour into a glass jar. Label and leave to set. Rub into rough patches and leave to soak in.

Storage: Keeps in an airtight jar for up to 3 months. **Dose:** Use as required.

MAKES
About 90g
(3¼oz)

JASMINE MORNING FACE MIST

A refreshing and hydrating mist with green tea that is high in antioxidants and antibacterials for combination skins. You will need a 100ml (3½fl oz/scant ½ cup) spray bottle – use an empty one from your wash bag if you can.

INGREDIENTS

~ 1 jasmine green tea bag

~ boiling water

~ 3 drops of vitamin E oil (or jojoba essential oil)

METHOD

Place the tea bag in a mug and fill the mug with boiling water. Allow to brew for 5 minutes, then remove the tea bag and leave to cool.

Pour 100 ml (3½fl oz/scant ½ cup) of the brewed tea into the spray bottle and add the vitamin E drops. Shake before use.

Storage: Stays fresh for up to 1 month.

Dose: Use after cleaning for a refreshing morning mist.

MAKES
About 100 ml
(3½fl oz/scant
½ cup)

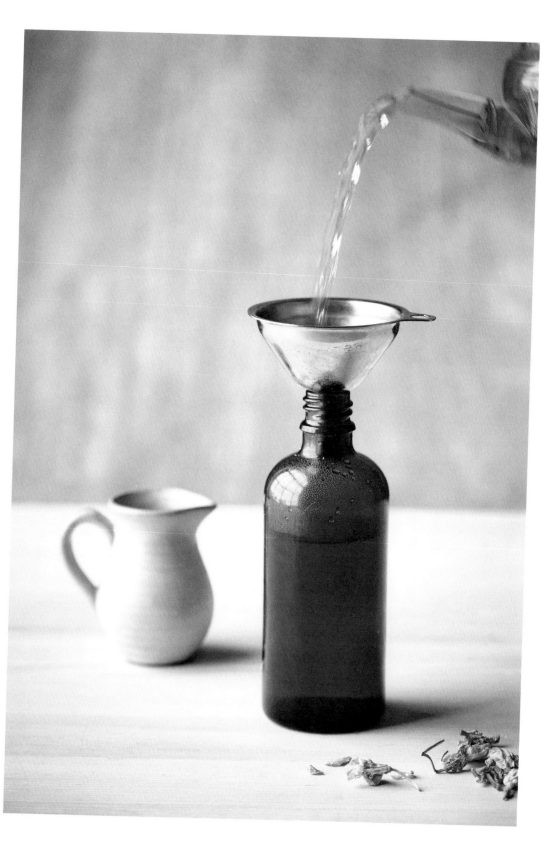

AVOCADO CREAM HYDRATION MASK

Rich and nourishing, this is a soothing and calming face mask that works for all skin types and is great for using up avocados. The vitamin A (retinol) can clear pores and reduce redness, while lecithin, a fatty acid, restores hydration. Studies have shown these can increase healing as well as reducing fine lines and wrinkles. You can tweak this to be a bespoke mask depending how your skin is feeling. Add a tablespoon of avocado oil to increase the richness for particularly thirsty skin or a tablespoon of yogurt for calming and cooling.

INGREDIENTS

~ 1 ripe avocado

~ 1 tsp raw honey

~ 1 tsp lemon juice

~ 1 tbsp avocado oil (optional)

~ 1 tbsp plain yogurt (optional)

METHOD

Scoop the avocado flesh into a bowl and mix until smooth.

Mix in the other ingredients, including the avocado oil for extra richness or the yogurt for extra calming.

Smooth onto the face, neck and décolletage and leave for 10 minutes.

Rinse off with water, pat dry with a towel and continue with your serums or toner and moisturiser as usual.

Storage: Use fresh as required.

Dose: Use once a week as required.

MAKES
One application

HIBISCUS SCALP TREATMENT FOR THINNING HAIR

Many reasons can be behind hair loss, sudden or gradual, so do look into these while you are trying to help bring your locks back to their fullness. Hibiscus has been used in shampoos, oils and hair treatments as a time-tested aid in helping to prevent hair loss, greyness and dandruff. This simple recipe is rich in flavonoids and amino acids that can help increase blood circulation to the scalp and revive dormant hair follicles, thereby stimulating new hair growth.

INGREDIENTS

~ 300g (10½oz) plain live yogurt

~ 1 tbsp hibiscus powder

METHOD

Combine the 2 ingredients in a bowl. Apply to damp hair from the scalp through to the ends, working it into the scalp well. Leave on for 1 hour.

Rinse and shampoo as usual.

Storage: Make fresh as required.

Dose: Use once a week as required.

TIP: Hibiscus powder is made from ground dried leaves and flowers and is available in health food stores.

MAKES
One application

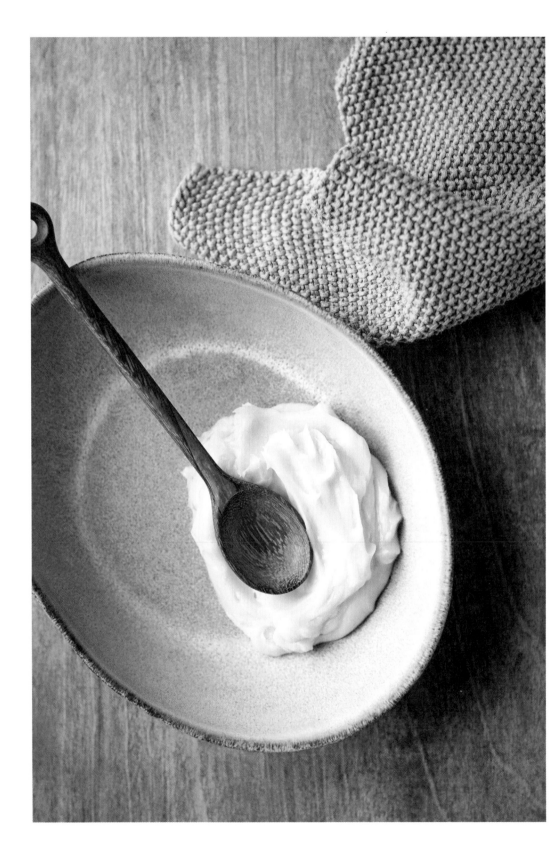

WHIPPED COCONUT & HONEY HAIR SHINE MASK

Adding lustre to hair shafts has regularly meant the use of plastics and ways of coating the hair to give an appearance of sheen, but with this entirely edible mask, the goodness is absorbed into the hair, providing it with real nourishment, strengthening and protecting it, and including antimicrobial goodness for scalp health and creating an incredible shine. The lauric acid content gives the roots protection as well as preventing hair breakage.

INGREDIENTS

~ 3 tbsp coconut oil

~ 2 tbsp raw honey

~ 1 tbsp apple cider vinegar

~ a few drops of essential oil (optional)

MAKES
About 90ml
(3fl oz/⅓ cup)

METHOD

Melt the coconut oil and stir into a jar with the honey and vinegar. If you find the vinegar too heady, add an essential oil to balance the smell. Whip it up with a hand-held blender to create a rich, creamy consistency.

Using your hands, smooth a handful of the cream through to ends of the hair, massaging into the scalp. Use a shower cap or tie the hair up and leave the ingredients to soak into the hair shafts for 15–30 minutes. If the hair is suffering from dryness, leave it on longer. Rinse and wash as normal.

Storage: Store in a glass jar in a cool, dark place for up to 2 months.

Dose: Use once a week.

CHARCOAL & COFFEE FACE SCRUB

One of the motivations for me in creating any of these lotions and potions was as much about using things that were bi-products of family life, such as coffee grounds, as replacing expensive jars with simple, natural ingredients. Upcycling your morning coffee to the mainstay of an evening facial feels smart, thrifty and luxurious all at once. The texture of the grinds with the absorption of the charcoal make this a fabulous exfoliator, and the coconut oil is healing and nourishing for any rough, dry skin.

INGREDIENTS

~ 1 tbsp coffee grinds, used and dried (or some prefer to use fresh)

~ ½ tbsp activated charcoal

~ 1 tbsp coconut oil

METHOD

Mix all the ingredients together in a small bowl. It is best to apply the scrub in the bath or shower as it can be a messy process. Smooth onto a dry face and rub gently. Wash off with water and cleanse as required.

Storage: Keeps in a dark glass jar in a cool, dry place for up to 3 months.

Dose: Use once a week or as needed for dry patches.

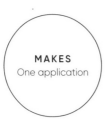

MAKES
One application

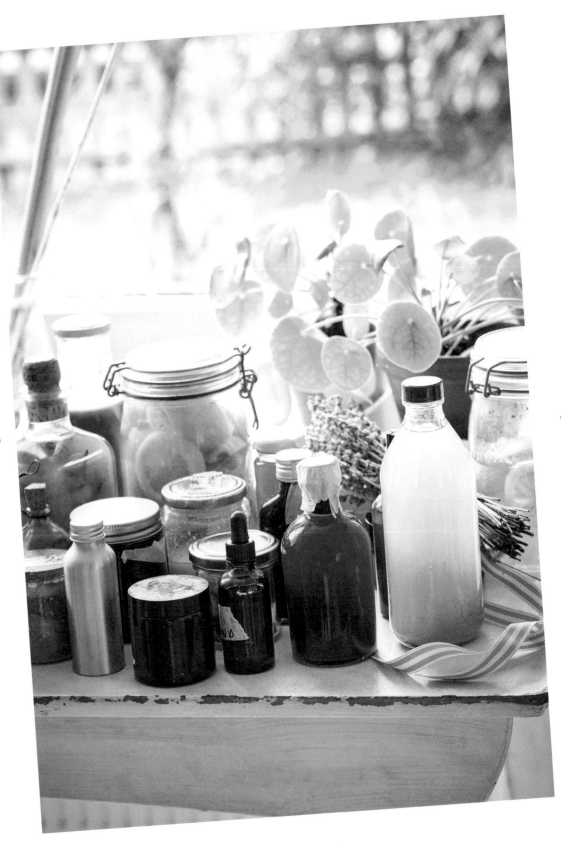

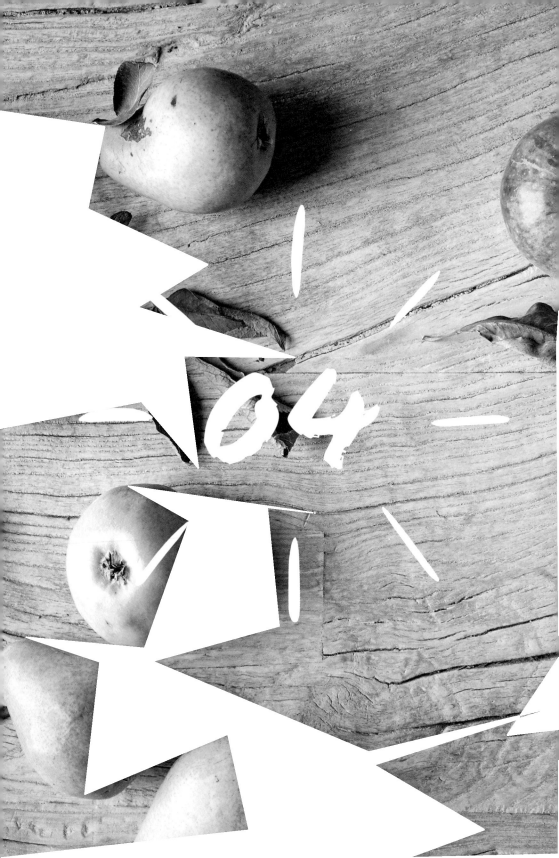

SHINE

I am not a naturally crafty, thrifty, make-your-own everything type. But I got into the idea of having some homemade cleaning potions to hand when looking at preserving gut health (and minimising antibacs).

The ingredients in common cleaning products made me switch up to greener options a while ago, but it wasn't until I was making body scrubs and bath oils that I saw how simple it could be, using mainly staple ingredients.

If we're avoiding pesticides and hormones in food – shown to have links with increased allergies, and some cancers – then it seemed out of whack to be pouring bleach and fierce antibacterial chemicals on everything we prep food on, eat with, touch and breathe in. Moreover, our skin and airways don't have the barriers our digestive system has, so any toxins absorbed go directly into our blood stream. I haven't come to this overnight, but the recipes all take minutes to make, definitely save pennies, and bring huge amounts of smug self-congratulation.

From the same joy of knowing exactly what you are eating and where it came from, there is much satisfaction knowing what you are spraying throughout the house in the name of hygiene, with ingredients you can lick off the kitchen table.

CLEANING NASTIES UNPACKED

Some of the ingredients used in everyday cleaning products are not things you would like to swallow or have in contact with your skin, yet this is what happens to household sprays and wipes. And in the same way we absorb unwanted chemicals from our food, we also breathe them in, absorb them through our skin or ingest them from our plates and kitchen surfaces. Watch out on the labels for some of the worst offenders so you can avoid them.

TRICLOSAN

An antibacterial and antifungal chlorine compound, it was banned by the FDA in 2016 from hand wash in the USA but remains in many products in the UK and elsewhere. Research has shown that it can cross the skin barrier and be found in urine and breast milk. It is linked to allergies in children and hormone disruption.

Risk: Can promote the growth of drug-resistant bacteria, increase allergies and disrupt hormones.

Found in: Hand wash, toothpaste and detergents.

Switch to: Natural antibacterial agents, such as lemon, vinegar, tea tree and eucalyptus oils.

PHTHALATES

These are compounds that add the scent to cleaning products but are not required to be in labelling, so are often just listed as 'fragrance'.

Risk: Known endocrine disruptors, the risk is from inhaling but also skin contact with soaps. Aerosol sprays and air fresheners can also be asthma and migraine triggers. A study in 2003 by Harvard Health found that men with higher phthalate readings had lower sperm counts.

Found in: Air fresheners, soaps, even toilet paper.

Switch to: Essential oils or natural scents from citrus and herbs, or choose fragrance-free.

PERCHLOROETHYLENE (PERC)

The most commonly used solvent in dry cleaning and stain removal, this is now banned in the USA.

Risk: A neurotoxin, perc has been named a 'probable human carcinogen'. It causes dizziness and is thought to be linked to cancers.

Found in: Dry cleaning solution, stain removers and carpet cleaners.

Switch to: 'Wet cleaning' that uses water-based options instead of solvents. For stain removing, rub undiluted castile liquid soap onto marks before washing.

TIP: Rebecca Sutton, PhD, says the risk with household cleaning products is that 'neither ingredients nor products must meet any sort of safety standard, nor is any testing data or notification required before bringing a product to market'.

THE TOXIC BURDEN

Manufacturers agree that these toxins in small doses are not likely to pose a problem, but frequent and long-term exposure and in unknown combinations makes it impossible to gauge the risks. The 'toxic body burden' is the chief concern surrounding household chemicals. Being exposed a handful of times to a chemical may not cause any harm, but chronic exposure daily, weekly or over a lifetime may cause a build-up or create enough damage to trigger a 'disease outcome'. As Sutton explains, 'the concept of body burden is that pollution is not just in our air and water – it's also in us.'

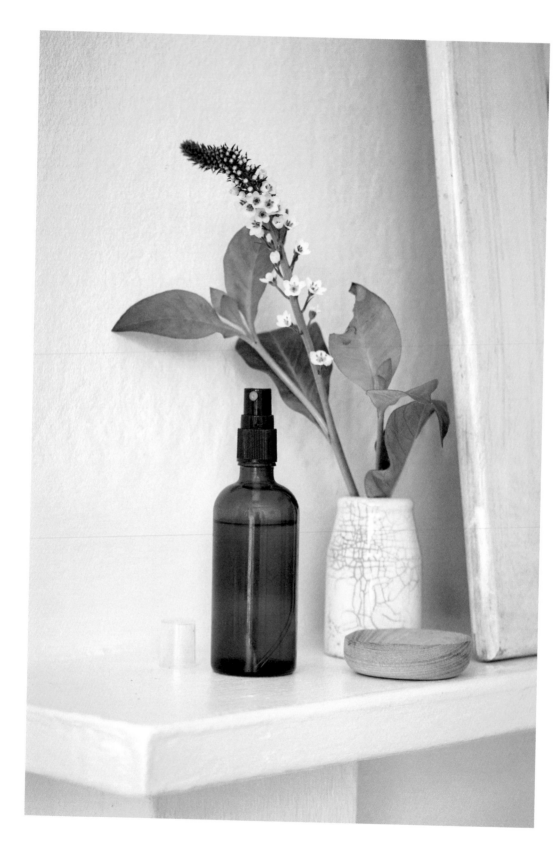

GERANIUM ROOM SPRAY

The leaves of this sunny flower are such an invocation of summer days. This freshens and brightens up a room, without filling it with the toxins that can be so harsh on the respiratory system. Play around with combinations, as once you start making these you'll use them for smelly sports kit, teenage bedrooms and anywhere else where you need the scent of summer. You will need a 100ml (3½fl oz/scant ½ cup) amber glass spray bottle.

INGREDIENTS

~ 15 drops of geranium essential oil

~ 5 drops of sandalwood essential oil

~ 1 tbsp witch hazel (or vodka)

~ filtered water

METHOD

Add everything to the spray bottle and top up with filtered water. Shake well.

Storage: Stays fresh for up to 6 months.

Dose: Use as needed.

MAKES
about 100 ml
(3½fl oz/scant
½ cup)

VASE DE-SLIMER

One of my first discoveries was how to use a few cupboard staples to get rid of the green slime that flower water creates without pouring bleach down the sink and round the kitchen. For the experts among you, it is indeed deemed a no-no combination, as the two chemicals used here cancel each other out, but the effervescent effect is brilliant at getting the green grot from inside vases and tricky-to-reach crannies.

INGREDIENTS

~ water

~ 1 tbsp bicarbonate of soda (baking soda)

~ 2 tbsp white vinegar, plus extra for wiping

~ 1 tsp sea salt flakes

MAKES
One application

METHOD

Pour enough water into the vase to come up to the tide mark. Add the bicarbonate of soda and then the vinegar and watch as the water begins to fizz and foam – a joy to watch. Once this has died down, dip a soft cloth into some vinegar and sprinkle the sea salt flakes over the top. Use this to work off any marks, which should come away easily.

Rinse, dry off and enjoy the sparkle!

Storage: Make as required.

Dose: Use as needed.

OLIVE OIL WOOD POLISH

This nourishes wood and brings out the shine, and also repairs shallow scratches brilliantly by soaking in and matching the colour of the rest of the wood. Many furniture polishes contain formaldehyde, paraffin and lists of ingredients you wouldn't want to inhale. This makes a pleasant change, using only regular olive oil and simple white vinegar.
Do not be tempted to replace the olive oil with other vegetable oils here – they don't do the job and they may damage the wood.

INGREDIENTS

~ 200ml (7fl oz/scant 1 cup) olive oil

~ 100ml (3½fl oz/scant ½ cup) white vinegar

METHOD

Mix the two ingredients together. Using a soft cloth, cotton or old tea towel, dip into the polish mix and wipe onto the wood, paying particular attention to scratches, working the polish into these until the marks virtually disappear. Leave to dry. Repeat if the wood still looks dull or dry.

Storage: Keeps for up to 6 months.

Dose: Use as required.

MAKES
About 300ml
(10½fl oz/scant
1¼ cups)

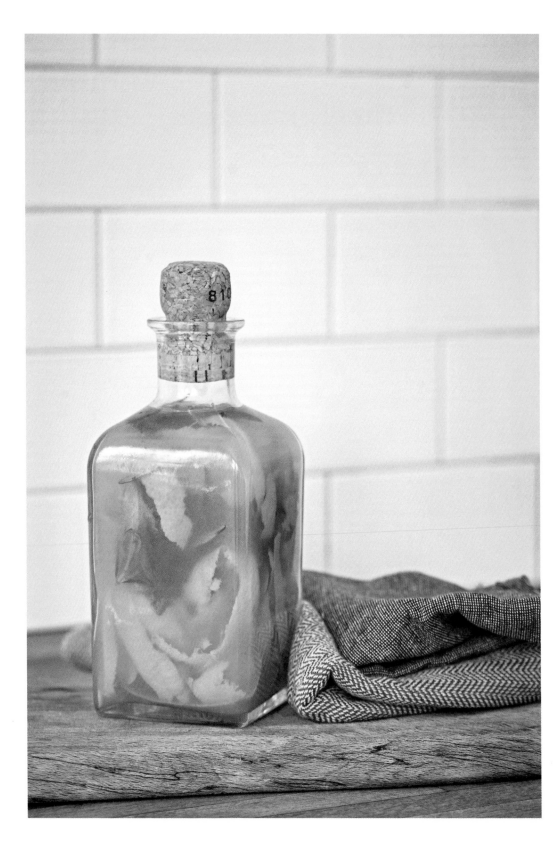

ZERO WASTE LEMON OIL KITCHEN SPRAY

This was my initiation recipe and the moment I realised that I loved making these concoctions. I was reading about vinegar – the most common DIY cleaner that goes in just about every single one out there – and I noted that you could also use the harsh acidity of it to draw the essential oils out of the lemon peels you were throwing away. The limonene that is produced is a powerful degreasing agent and it turns into a multi-purpose addition to any solution where vinegar could be used, with extra oomph. As a cook, and habitual lemon tea drinker, I get through so many that the empty peels pile up. Now I put them to good use by dropping them in a jar of vinegar and steeping for a couple of weeks. You are left with a deliciously astringent lemon oil concentrate that you can add to water or include in another recipe instead of vinegar. It does an amazing job without the vinegar.

INGREDIENTS

~ 400ml (13fl oz/generous 1½ cups) white vinegar

~ 1 sprig of rosemary (or thyme) (optional)

~ juice of 5–6 lemons

~ cooled boiled water

METHOD

Pour the vinegar into a 1 litre (34fl oz/4 cup) Kilner (Mason) jar; it will come up to about the halfway mark. Add the herbs, if using. As you use up lemons in cooking, tea or drinks, add the rinds to the jar, pushing them below the liquid level. Leave in a cool, dark spot in your kitchen for 2 weeks.

Strain the liquid into a measuring jug, discarding the lemon peeld and herb sprigs, and dilute in a 50/50 ratio with cooled boiled water. Pour into a spray bottle and use on all kitchen grime on surfaces and pans, tough greasy hob marks, baking trays and anything else.

Storage: Keeps for about 6 months.

Dose: Use as needed.

TIP: Please note that this is not to be used on marble, granite or stoneware as it can cause discoloration.

MAKES
About 1 litre
(34fl oz/4 cups)

INSTANT SINK UNBLOCKER

More amateur chemistry fun than domestic chore, this fizzes and bubbles
and creates an incredible froth that ends with a burp effect, and hopefully
a spotless U-bend under your sink without any elbow grease involved.

INGREDIENTS

~ 200g (7oz/scant 1 cup) bicarbonate
of soda (baking soda)

~ 300ml (10½fl oz/scant 1¼ cups)
white vinegar

~ 300ml (10½fl oz/scant 1¼ cups)
cooled boiled water

~ 2 kettles of boiling water

METHOD

Boil the kettle and pour the contents into the blocked sink
hole. Carefully tip in the bicarbonate of soda, trying
to get as much into the sink hole as possible. Mix the
vinegar and measured water together in a small jug, then
pour it into the sink and put the plug in while the
chemicals get to work for 5 minutes.

Boil another kettle and pour this in next. You should
find some dramatic burping and fizzing and an ensuing
cleaned-out sink.

Storage: Make fresh as required.

Dose: Repeat as necessary.

MAKES
One application

FRESH & BRIGHTENING ROOM SPRAY

Having always shunned plug-in room fresheners both for the smells they give off and the ingredients within, I've relied on candles or open windows to refresh a room. But now I am adding this gentle spray to lift a room at the beginning of the day, before someone arrives or after a good clean up. It's a lovely addition to the home, and again you can tweak as you like.

INGREDIENTS

~ 1 tbsp witch hazel (or vodka)

~ 10 drops of geranium essential oil

~ 5 drops of lemon essential oil

~ 5 drops of orange essential oil

~ 100ml (3½fl oz/scant ½ cup) cooled boiled water

METHOD

Add the witch hazel or alcohol and essential oils to a small spray bottle, fill with water and screw on the spray nozzle. Label (not forgetting to date it) and store in a dark cupboard.

To use, spritz into the room that requires refreshing, or spritz the air as you walk into it for an instant mood lift.

Storage: Keeps in a cool, dark place for up to 6 months.

Dose: Use as required.

TIP: Adding plants to your home is a natural air detoxifier; they purify air as they mop up CO_2 and fill up your home with clean oxygen.

MAKES
About 120ml
(4fl oz/scant
½ cup)

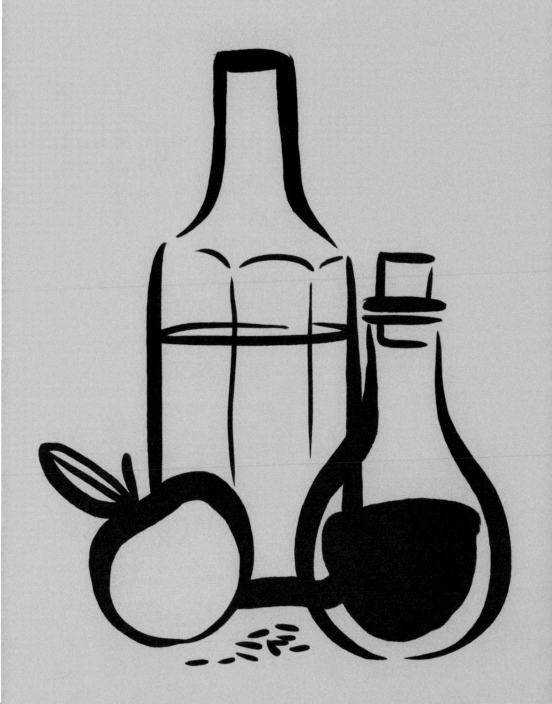

SPOTLIGHT ON
VINEGAR

Vinegar has been used by our ancestors as both a condiment and preservative as far back as the Babylonians in 5000BCE and in the urns of the Egyptians from 3000BCE. Its use as a remedy has been documented for almost as long. The Ancient Greek physician Hippocrates, in 400BCE, prescribed vinegar for ailments from skin rashes to ear infections. We all know the nursery rhyme in which Jack goes to bed to mend his head 'with vinegar and brown paper'.

Made by fermenting diluted alcohol products with various fruits and grains, yielding the organic compound acetic acid, vinegar is one of the oldest and most versatile elements to any remedies. Used from the kitchen counter to the medicine cabinet, as well as a culinary accent, its acetic acid properties are what provide its preserving, cleansing, blood-sugar-balancing and antiseptic qualities.

The word 'vinegar' came from the Latin for sour wine (*vinum acer*) and the first vinegars were probably created from mistakes in the wine-making process. It was used to preserve foods that needed transportation, enjoyed as a 'poor man's' wine, and was commonly used as a herbicide and in folk remedies. Its unique chemical make-up was not fully understood until Louis Pasteur's study 'Etudes sur le Vinaigre' in 1858.

As its popularity increased, so has its practical applications for culinary, medicinal and sanitary purposes. Proven to work effectively as a herbicide on crops, and to lower the glycaemic index when taken before eating, vinegar remains an effective, easy-to-come-by and inexpensive addition to a natural remedy resource.

EUCALYPTUS BATHROOM CLEANER

Where we spend hours washing, relaxing, inhaling and soaking should be the place to start when we know how much is absorbed through our skin. This delightful cleaner smells like a walk in a forest, works a treat and has antibacterial properties to keep the bathroom clean in a gentler way. I never thought I'd be a make-your-own bath spray person, to be honest, and cleaning is not a task that has ever excited me, but the act of creating them and adoring them makes it all so much more enjoyable. There's joy in the sheer simplicity of putting a few things (that you love) into a bottle and fiddling with the smell until you are happy.

INGREDIENTS

~ 500ml (17 fl oz/2 cups) boiled water, cooled to lukewarm

~ 1 tbsp bicarbonate of soda (baking soda)

~ 2 tsp castile liquid soap

~ 2 tbsp eucalyptus essential oil

METHOD

Pour the water into a measuring jug and add the remaining ingredients. Stir well to dissolve. Using lukewarm water will make it easier to mix the ingredients.

Funnel into a spray bottle and you're ready to sparkle.

Storage: Keeps indefinitely.

Dose: Use as required.

MAKES
About 500ml
(17 fl oz/2 cups)

GLASS & MIRROR SPARKLE SPRAY

There are single-ingredient ways of wiping the grime off windows that work well, but I found the combination here meant that the smearing and smudges were dealt with too. The alcohol content means it evaporates quickly and without any sweat, glass and mirrors will look gleaming.

INGREDIENTS

~ 400ml (13fl oz/generous 1½ cups) water, freshly boiled

~ 2 tbsp vodka (or witch hazel)

~ 2 tbsp white vinegar

~ 15 drops of neroli essential oil (or use grapefruit or another citrus essential oil)

METHOD

Pour the ingredients into a spray bottle, shake to mix, and label.

Shake well before each use, spray onto glass or mirror surface and, using a clean, soft cloth, sweep across in a circular motion. Follow up with a clean, dry, lint-free cloth to buffer the cleaned area and let it shine.

Storage: Keeps indefinitely.

Dose: Use as required.

MAKES
About 450ml
(15¾fl oz/
scant 2 cups)

GRAPEFRUIT LOO RINSE

One of the areas that often remain bleach-heavy, the toilet bowl can be a harder graft to clean when using less-than-industrial-strength products. Although no one is coming too close to this chinaware, the fumes from the chlorine gases that bleaches create can affect us, irritating eyes, noses and throats and aggravating the respiratory system generally. This is a decent and much kinder solution.

INGREDIENTS

~ 200ml (7fl oz/scant 1 cup) water

~ 100g (3½oz/scant ½ cup) bicarbonate of soda (baking soda)

~ 100ml (3½fl oz/scant ½ cup) castile liquid soap

~ 2 tbsp grapefruit essential oil

~ white vinegar, to spray

METHOD

Pour the water and bicarbonate of soda into a spray bottle and stir to dissolve. Add the soap and oil, and mix together well.

To use, spray the toilet bowl with the mixture, and using neat white vinegar in a spray bottle of its own, spray on top and leave to sit for 5–10 minutes before flushing to rinse.

Storage: Keeps for up to 6 months.

Dose: Use as required.

MAKES
About 400ml
(13fl oz/generous
1½ cups)

YLANG YLANG LOO SPRAY

Small rooms that are used frequently can become pungent fast, so they need efficient ways of freshening up. I love this floral relief that seems to dissipate most smells quickly.

INGREDIENTS

~ 1 tbsp alcohol (see Tip) or witch hazel

~ 2 tbsp ylang ylang essential oil

~ 5 drops of grapefruit essential oil

~ 100ml (3½fl oz/scant ½ cup) water

METHOD

Add the witch hazel or alcohol to a small spray bottle and mix in the essential oils. Top up with water and shake.

Label 'Please Use Loo Spray' and leave on the side by the cistern to encourage its use and help your loo to stay fresh.

Storage: Keeps for up to 6 months.

Dose: Use regularly as required.

TIP: Try budget 35% vodka.

MAKES
About 120ml
(4fl oz/scant
¼ cup)

ORANGE & LEMON ALL-SURFACE LICKABLE SPRAY

Where you cook and eat, and the kids play, is often wiped more than any other place in the house, and often this is with a cocktail of chemicals and things you wouldn't want near your children's delicate skin and lungs. By putting together a bottle of food-grade goodness yourself, you can keep the surfaces clean and the germs away with a delicious smell you can tweak as desired. This does well to wipe everything from kitchen tables, to walls, to desks. You'll need a spray bottle, so re-use one from the kitchen.

INGREDIENTS

~ 10 drops of lemon essential oil

~ 10 drops of orange essential oil

~ 3 tbsp castile liquid soap

~ 500ml (17fl oz/2 cups) water

METHOD

Mix the oils and soap with the water in a spray bottle. Shake before use.

Storage: Keeps indefinitely.

Dose: Shake before using whenever you like.

TIP: Unlike the vinegar-based cleaners, this can also be used on granite and stoneware.

MAKES
About 500ml
(178fl oz/2 cups)

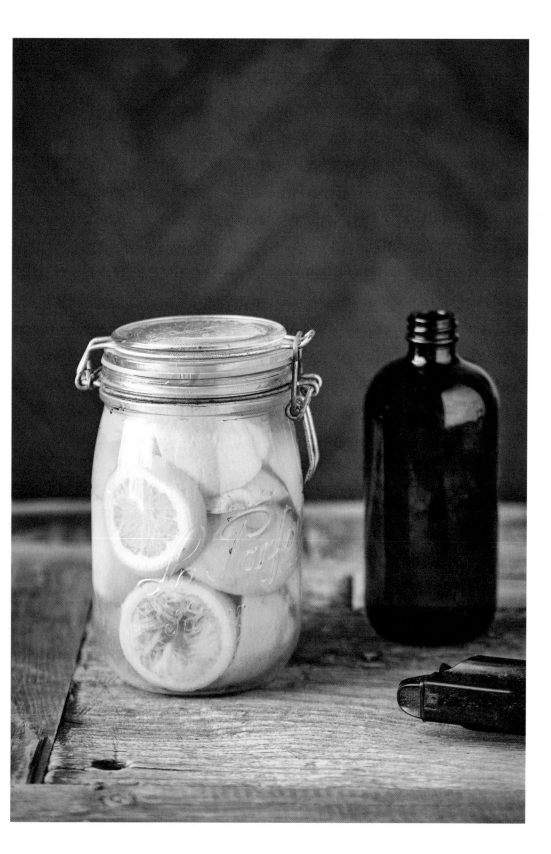

BLOOD, MUD & WINE STAIN REMOVER

Harsh stain removers are one of the worst perpetrators when it comes to skin irritation and potential respiratory damage, and these household ingredients work so beautifully there is no need to keep the industrial-grade ones in the house. Another case of simple chemical reactions at work, the components of these common family stains mean matching them up with the most effective method of extraction.

Berries: Apply neat lemon juice to the stain and rub gently.

Blood: Mix equal quantities of white vinegar and cold water, leave to soak for 30 minutes, then wash.

Mud: Rinse well with water and then apply a spoonful of bicarbonate of soda (baking soda) and leave to

soak for 30 minutes. Rinse, rubbing with more bicarbonate of soda for any stubborn marks.

Wine: Sprinkle sea salt flakes onto the wet stain to lift the first marks. Make a paste of equal parts of

bicarbonate of soda and water, leave to soak for 2 hours, then rinse and wash as normal

Storage: Use fresh as required. **Dose:** Use as required.

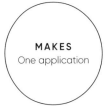

MAKES
One application

JEWELLERY SPARKLE SOAKS

As a constant jewellery wearer – I sleep, swim and shower in the same set of everything – the sparkle can dim and the residue of creams and life needs cleaning off once in a while. With these options, there's no need to go to the professionals to restore your shine. The first is a catch-all for most metals and stones, and the second option works particularly beautifully for silver and diamonds. Do be careful where you put this glass full of preciousness as you do NOT want anyone to throw this away by mistake.

ALL-METAL SHINE SOAK

INGREDIENTS ~ boiling water ~ squirt of castile liquid soap

METHOD Put your jewellery in a mug or dish and pour over enough boiling water to cover. Add a squirt of liquid soap, mix and leave to soak for 30 minutes. Use a soft toothbrush to clean thoroughly. Rinse and leave to dry. **Storage:** Make fresh as required. **Dose:** As often as you like.

SILVER & DIAMOND SOAK

INGREDIENTS ~ 100ml (3½fl oz/scant ½ cup) white vinegar

~ 1 tbsp bicarbonate of soda (baking soda)

METHOD Put your jewellery in a mug or dish, add the vinegar, then sprinkle over the bicarbonate of soda. Leave to soak for 1–2 hours. Use a toothbrush to remove any lodged-in dirt. Rinse and leave to dry. **Storage:** Make fresh as required. **Dose:** As often as you like.

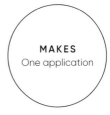

MAKES
One application

LAVENDER FLOOR WASH

Here's another way to re-use those spray bottles in the kitchen you won't need any more! This brings the delightful scent of lavender as well as its antibacterial properties.

INGREDIENTS

~ 100ml (3½fl oz/scant ½ cup) white vinegar

~ 100ml (3½fl oz/scant ½ cup) vodka or clear alcohol (or witch hazel)

~ 15 drops of lavender essential oil

~ 4 drops of castile liquid soap

~ 200ml (7fl oz/scant 1 cup) filtered water

METHOD

In a large spray bottle, combine the vinegar and alcohol or witch hazel. Drop in the oil and liquid soap, then top up with water. Stir with a wooden spoon handle to combine or put on the lid and shake well.

Storage: Keeps for up to 6 months.

Dose: Shake before using whenever you like.

MAKES
About 400ml
(13fl oz/generous
1½ cups)

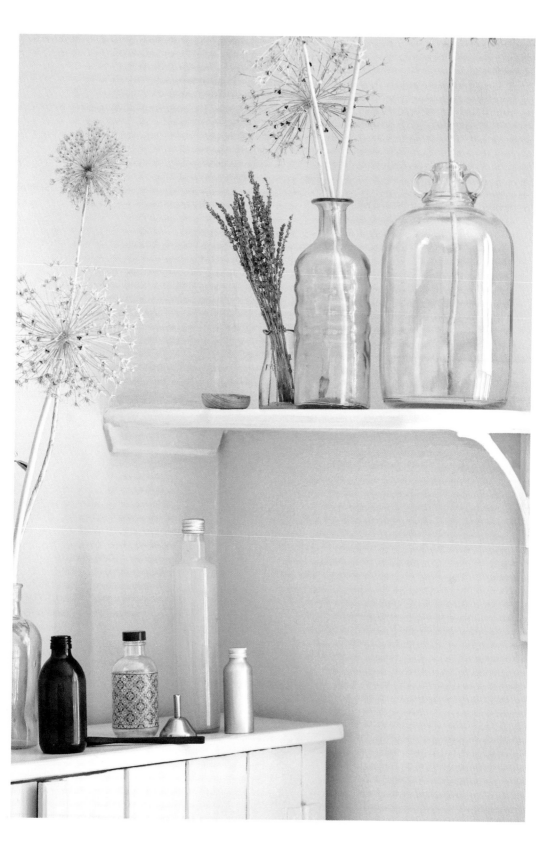

SODA KETTLE DESCALER

The joy of this instant kettle cleaner is that you can see it at work. The build-up of limescale means unwanted additions to your cuppas, but also makes the kettle less efficient, as it uses more electricity to heat through the muffling effects of the limescale, so this is an energy saver as well as a satisfying clean-up tool. For the hardest-working machine in anyone's house, it will last longer and more effectively if you show it some love now and again.

INGREDIENTS

~ 2 tbsp bicarbonate of soda (baking soda)

~ water

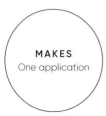

MAKES
One application

METHOD

Fill the kettle to just over halfway and add the bicarbonate of soda. Switch the kettle on to boil, remove the lid and watch the effervescent cleaning at work. Leave to sit for an hour, then rinse well. Repeat if any limescale remains.

This can be done as often as you like, depending on water hardness and how much you use the kettle.

Storage: Make as needed.

Dose: Every 3 months or more frequently in hard-water areas.

TIP: To descale your washing machine, pour 700ml (24fl oz/2¾ cups) of white vinegar into the main drum of the machine and run on the hottest wash. Once finished, repeat but using 400g (14oz/heaped 1¾ cups) of bicarbonate of soda (baking soda).

PARSLEY BREATH FRESHENER

Bad breath, or halitosis, can be a result of underlying health or dental conditions, dietary or digestive issues, or just a one-off. Whichever it is, it is something that anyone who suffers from it or lives with someone who can be prone to it would love to resolve. Vinegar is a great start as an all-round antibacterial mouthwash. Parsley is high in the green pigment chlorophyll, which is both neutralising and deodorising. This is particularly effective as an instant cure for garlic breath – the stems neutralise the sulphuric compounds of the garlic.

INGREDIENTS

~ 1 tbsp apple cider vinegar

~ 1 tbsp water

~ 1 tbsp chopped parsley leaves and stems

METHOD

Simply mix together the vinegar and water and rinse around your mouth for a few seconds, spit and repeat until the mouth feels fresh. Finally, chew on the fresh parsley for a minute or two.

Storage: Make fresh as required.

Dose: Use once a day or as needed.

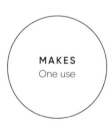

MAKES
One use

WOODEN CHOPPING BOARD STAIN SCRUB

I'm a die-hard wooden chopping board fan – I love them as serving boards, as well as preferring them to work on by far to the feel of plastic. Plastic is often touted as a more hygienic option, but happily it has now been shown that wood is inherently antibacterial; the natural cellulose actively destroys both surface and embedded bacteria. As a further plus, they are kinder to knives. But they can stain and need a spruce up or an odour reliever – and this one is so simple.

INGREDIENTS

~ 115g (4oz/½ cup) bicarbonate of soda (baking soda)

~ 1 lemon, halved

~ hot water

METHOD

Sluice the board down of any debris under the tap and shake off any excess water.

Sprinkle over the bicarbonate of soda and leave for a couple of minutes; it will fizz slightly. Then, using the lemon halves, work the soda into the surface whilst squeezing the juice at the same time and covering the whole board. Leave for 10 minutes, then rinse well with warm water and dry.

Storage: Make fresh as required.

Dose: Use whenever your board is stained or needs to be refreshed.

MAKES
One application

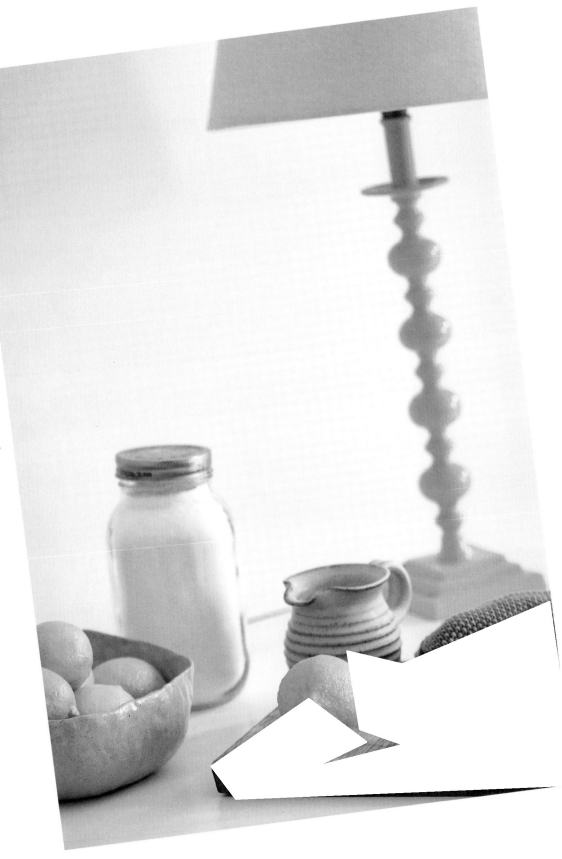

CITRUS OVEN DE-GREASER

Undoubtedly the least favourite task in the house, this often gets neglected, and in the main because it feels impossible to make a dent in the dark grease caked onto the oven, unless there is a vicious cocktail of neon-coloured creams involved. The beauty and power of citric acid comes into its own here, and the crunchy baked zest means the natural exfoliating properties combine with the chemical grease-stripping acids to give a deliciously effective rub.

INGREDIENTS

~ 1 grapefruit

~ 1 orange

~ 3 tbsp bicarbonate of soda (baking soda)

~ 4 tbsp coarse sea salt

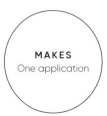

MAKES
One application

METHOD

Preheat the oven to 160°C (320°F/gas 3) and line a baking sheet with baking parchment.

Peel the zest from the grapefruit and the orange with a potato peeler in thick strips, keeping it in as few pieces as possible. Spread it over the baking sheet and bake for 10–15 minutes, or until it is looking dry but not browning at the edges. Leave until cool enough to touch, then crush to a coarse powder in a pestle and mortar.

Combine the soda, salt and citrus zest in a small bowl. Spritz the inside of your oven with water, then scatter the mixture over the damp oven and leave for 20–30 minutes. With a small brush, scrub to remove the grease, then rinse to clean. Repeat as necessary. For more ingrained dirt, leave on overnight.

Storage: Make as required.

Dose: Regularly.

TIP: Add a handful of sea salt and a generous glug of olive oil to any cast-iron pans that have burnt-on food and leave to sit for at least 1 hour. Scrub with a small brush and keep adding salt and oil until clean.

LIME REFRIGERATOR FRESHENER

No one is immune to a case of refrigerator stench! Seeping jars and leaking milk bottles can create a killer combination, and this simple addition to the shelves can help keep these smells at bay. Here, the citrus works as a deodoriser. You need to start with a clean refrigerator, so have a clear out and a wipe down to make this worthwhile.

INGREDIENTS

~ 2 limes or lemons

MAKES
One application

METHOD

Cut the limes or lemons in half and juice them. Pour the juice into a small jar and add the cut fruit halves too. Place on the shelf in the refrigerator. This needs to be changed once a month.

Storage: Keep in the back of the refrigerator.

Dose: Effective for up to a month.

TIP: To freshen up your dishwasher, add any used lemon halves to the top rack and it will add extra cleaning power and fragrance to your wash. Change every use.

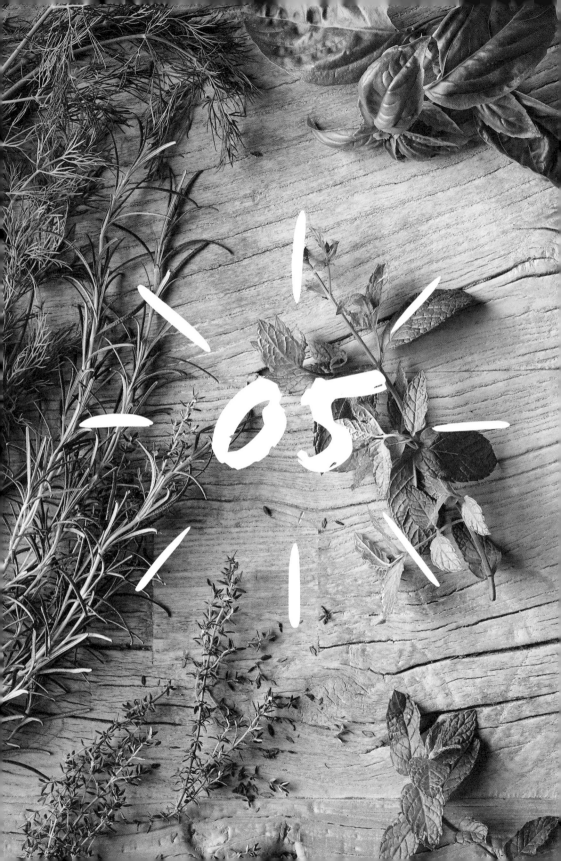

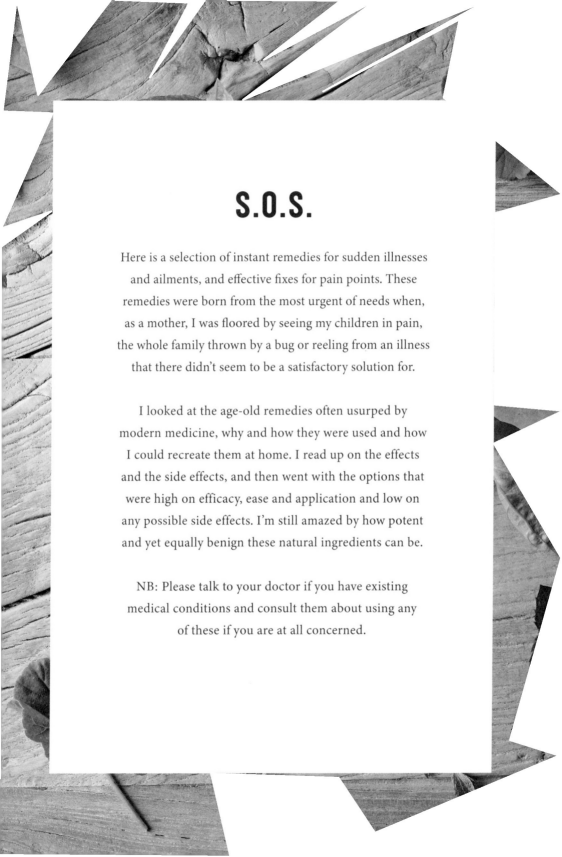

S.O.S.

Here is a selection of instant remedies for sudden illnesses and ailments, and effective fixes for pain points. These remedies were born from the most urgent of needs when, as a mother, I was floored by seeing my children in pain, the whole family thrown by a bug or reeling from an illness that there didn't seem to be a satisfactory solution for.

I looked at the age-old remedies often usurped by modern medicine, why and how they were used and how I could recreate them at home. I read up on the effects and the side effects, and then went with the options that were high on efficacy, ease and application and low on any possible side effects. I'm still amazed by how potent and yet equally benign these natural ingredients can be.

NB: Please talk to your doctor if you have existing medical conditions and consult them about using any of these if you are at all concerned.

HAY FEVER SUNSHINE SMOOTHIE

The natural antihistamine of bromelain and quercetin in pineapple work so well together here with the citrus vitamin C and the extra power from the reishi mushroom, which reduces antibody response and works to ease the sniffling, eye-watering and itching of allergy season.

INGREDIENTS

~ 210g (7½oz/1 cup) peeled and chopped pineapple (core included)

~ 1 frozen banana

~ juice of 1 orange

~ 1 tsp reishi mushroom powder

~ 250ml (9fl oz/generous 1 cup) milk of choice

METHOD

Blend together all the ingredients in a powerful food processor until evenly blended. Pour into a glass and serve immediately. Alternatively, freeze in large ice-cube trays, then pop them into freezer bags (they'll take up less room) and have whenever you need them. You can even serve them as lollies when the summer heat is all too much.

Storage: Freeze for up to 3 months.

Dose: Use as needed.

MAKES
About 540g
(1lb 3oz)

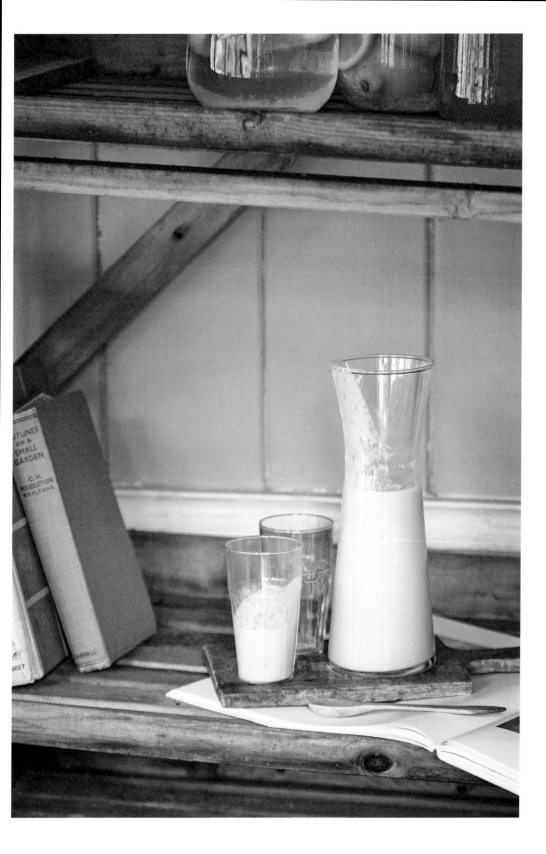

MAGNESIUM HEADACHE TONIC

Tension headaches and migraines are one of the most common reasons for a visit to the doctor, and I see the debilitation they can cause. While the simplest respite can be found in a large glass of water, there are longer-term lifestyle tweaks that might help individuals. For example, reducing stress levels and caffeine intake. Magnesium has been shown to alleviate the tension and constriction that can cause headaches, and this magnesium-rich drink was designed to bring relief.

INGREDIENTS

~ juice of 2 grapefruits

~ 1 handful of spinach leaves
(frozen works too)

~ 2 tbsp pumpkin seeds

~ handful of ice cubes

METHOD

Blend all ingredients together in a high-speed blender for 2–3 minutes. Drink immediately.

Storage: Make fresh as required.

Dose: Use daily as needed.

TIP: Migraine relief can be found by creating a stronger magnesium tonic by gently mixing 2 tablespoons of magnesium citrate with warm water, being careful that the mixture does not fizz out of the glass. Drink immediately and rest.

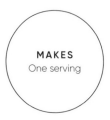

MAKES
One serving

TUMMY ACHE SOOTHING RICE SOCK

A sock full of rice is one of the simplest ideas I came across whilst researching this book and looking at ways of relieving tummy pains. It creates a damp heat rather than a dry one, and so is also really effective for muscular aches, with a useful shape for necks, lower backs and knees.

INGREDIENTS

~ 1 large thermal sock

~ 1kg (2lb 4oz/5 cups) uncooked white rice

MAKES
One reusable
sock

METHOD

Place the sock inside a vase or jug and fold the top over the edges of it. Pour in enough rice until the sock is three-quarters full. Tie to close, or sew shut if you prefer.

Heat the oven to 160°C (320°F/gas 3). Place the sock in a large casserole dish on the top shelf of the oven, with a second dish full of water below, to increase the humidity and prevent burning. Heat for 20–30 minutes, checking occasionally on the sock temperature. It should be warm to the touch but not too hot to handle.

Curl up with the warm sock on your tummy to relieve aches and pains.

Storage: Keep in a dry place for up to 3 months.

Dose: Use as required.

TIP: This doubles as an ice pack simply by placing it in the freezer.

ECZEMA HAND & BODY CREAM

Rough, red hands caused by harsh washing soaps or raw eczema patches can be hard to combat without resorting to brutal, skin-thinning hydrocortisone treatments. Oats are an emollient and also soothe any itching. For the porridge lovers, it's an extra joy that breakfast can be one of the healing ingredients.

INGREDIENTS

~ 200g (7oz/scant 1⅔ cups) oatmeal

~ 2 tbsp olive oil

~ 200ml (7fl oz/scant 1 cup) coconut oil

~ 5 drops rosemary essential oil (or use 1 sprig of rosemary, finely chopped)

METHOD

Put the oats (and rosemary if using fresh) into a powerful blender and grind to a powder. Add the olive oil and coconut oil and pulse until warmed up and thinning. Add the rosemary oil and blend until combined. Pour into a jar with a lid and let it cool until solid.

Use on any dry skin, eczema or itchy patches.

Storage: Stays fresh for up to 3–6 months.

Dose: Use as required.

MAKES
About
400g (14oz)

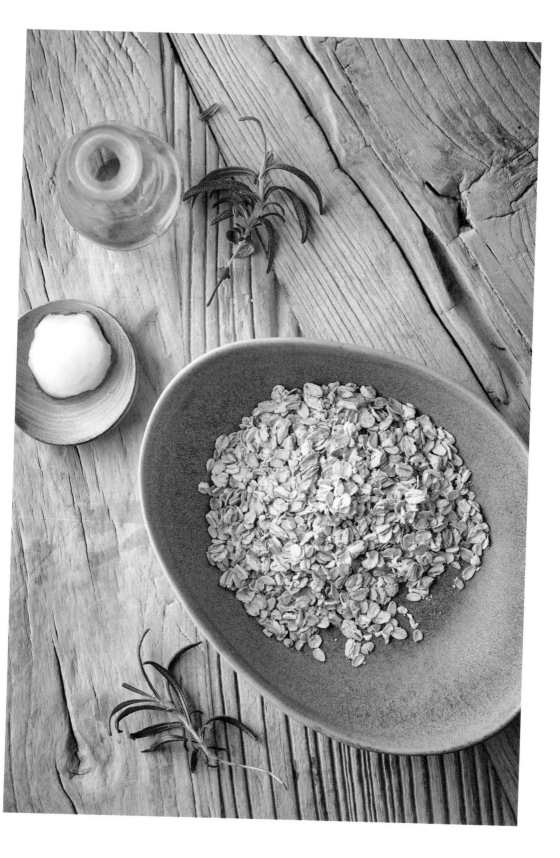

HAY FEVER NOSE BALM

The mechanical barrier option is so often more effective than other methods. and here the pollen is trapped before it enters the nostrils, making you less in need of chemical extras to function well. As is the case so often with natural remedies, it comes with zero side effects and can only make skin softer as a possible added extra.

INGREDIENTS

~ 1 tbsp coconut oil

~ 1 tbsp beeswax pellets

~ 4 drops of lemon essential oil

~ 3 drops of lavender essential oil

METHOD

In a heatproof bowl over boiling water, melt the coconut oil and beeswax pellets. Remove from the heat and stir in the oils. Pour into a jar while still warm. Leave to cool and add the lid once hardened.

Apply to the nostrils when needed.

Storage: Keep in an airtight jar for up to 3 months.

Dose: Use enough to rub into the outside of the nostrils as often as needed.

MAKES
About 30ml
(2 tbsp)

C.C.F. HEARTBURN TONIC

A favourite in Ayurveda, so fêted it is known by the acronym of the spice initials, the ingredients are easily found in your spice rack. This calming tea has been a night-time craving of mine since I came across it recently. It has a gently aromatic flavour and always helps if we have eaten too late or too richly.

INGREDIENTS

~ 1 tsp cumin seeds

~ 1 tsp coriander seeds

~ 1 tsp fennel seeds

~ 1 litre (34fl oz/4 cups) boiling water

METHOD

Add the spices to large tea pot and cover with just-boiled water. Leave to steep for 5 minutes.

Drink as many mugs as you like before bed, or when feeling the effects of heartburn or indigestion.

Storage: Make fresh as required.

Dose: Drink as much as you like as needed.

MAKES
About 1 litre
(34fl oz/4 cups)

WHIPPED MAGNESIUM BODY BUTTER

This unctuous, nourishing balm is a step beyond a skin smoother. It has helped me so much with helping getting a restful night's sleep and has eased the twitchy legs that I often suffer from. Many of us are lacking sufficient levels of magnesium, which impacts our ability to rest and relax. Applying magnesium through the skin (transdermal) can be a much more effective way of absorbing it into the blood stream rather than through the digestive system.

INGREDIENTS

~ 100g (3½oz/scant ½ cup) magnesium flakes

~ 2 tbsp boiling water

~ 3 tbsp shea butter

~ 2 tbsp beeswax pellets

~ 2 tbsp coconut oil

~ 10 drops of essential geranium oil (optional)

METHOD

Place the magnesium flakes in a mug and add 2 tablespoons of the boiling water, stirring to dissolve. Place the shea butter, beeswax pellets and coconut oil in a large, heatproof glass jar in a small pan of boiling water and leave to melt. Add the magnesium liquid and, using a hand-held blender, blend well to form a smooth butter. Pour into a glass jar and leave to cool and harden. Seal and label.

Use all over your body after an evening bath, sip a bedtime tea while it absorbs and retire to bed feeling blissfully relaxed for a heavenly night's sleep.

Storage: Stays fresh for up to 3 months.

Dose: Use as needed.

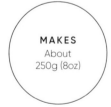

MAKES
About
250g (8oz)

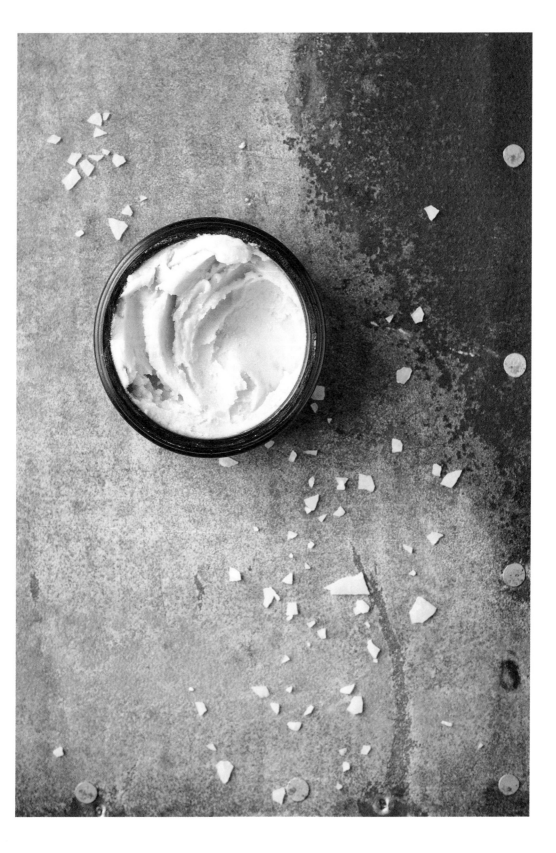

HONEY COUGH REMEDY

Cough syrups were a staple of my childhood, but when I read the labels and noted the sheer stickiness of them, I never thought they were doing much good. While raw honey has shone brightly as a time-honoured natural remedy for sore throats and coughs because of its antimicrobial and anti-inflammatory properties, I was particularly thrilled when the NHS recently recommended honey as the most effective cough relief for children. They even suggest it might be more effective than over-the-counter cough suppressants.

INGREDIENTS

~ 1–2 tsp raw honey

METHOD

Take an hour before bedtime to soothe coughs.

Storage: Keep honey in an airtight jar in a dark place.

Dose: Daily as needed.

TIP: I use Jarrah honey for its caramel flavour and active antimicrobials (the TA number on jars of honey denotes level of antimicrobial activity).

NOTE: Honey is not suitable for children under 1 year.

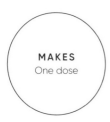

MAKES
One dose

NIT TREATMENT

Every parent of young children knows that heart-sinking feeling when their child comes home exhibiting the familiar relentless head scratching and an investigation reveals the discovery of nits. In store is the familiar cycle of evenings resigned to the yelling and hair-tugging and dousing of children that this inevitably means. For years we bought the recommended treatments, duly applied them and seemed never to be rid of the pestilent lice, or the revolting stench and oil slicks the treatments left us with. I have searched and trialled high and low in the name of easy, nit-free life, and with this potion, you can enjoy it too.

INGREDIENTS

~ 3 tbsp coconut oil

~ 1 tsp anise essential oil

~ ½ tsp ylang ylang essential oil

~ ½ tsp tea tree essential oil

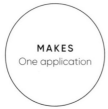

MAKES
One application

METHOD

In a large jar or mixing bowl, blend together the coconut oil and essential oils. You can use a hand-held blender for this for a speedier blend.

Apply to dry hair, massage into the scalp well and comb to the ends for full coverage.

Using a fine-toothed nit comb, section off the hair and comb through thoroughly. Much of the success depends on the thoroughness of this mechanical removal part of the process.

Rinse well, shampoo and condition as normal.

Storage: Make fresh as required.

Dose: Repeat every 5 days until you are nit-free.

TIP: One reassuring fact you should know is that nits actually like clean hair, so don't beat yourself up on that score!

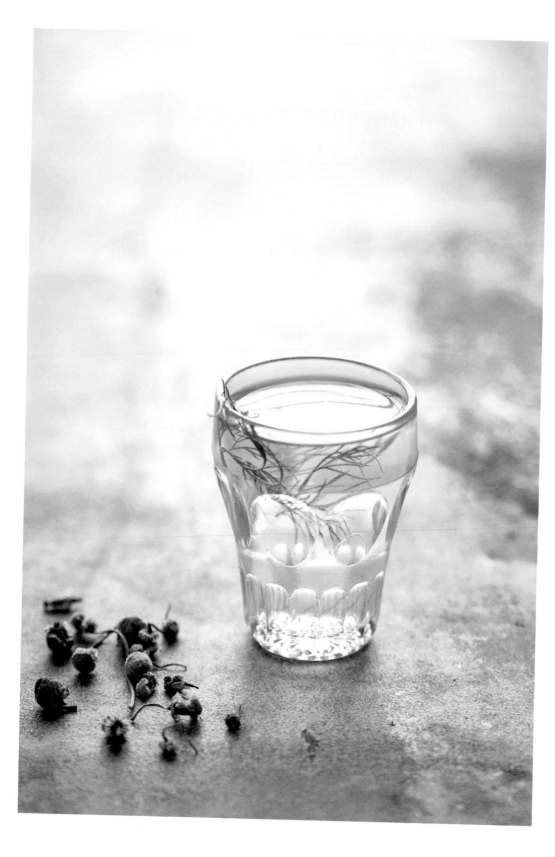

CHAMOMILE & DILL COLIC TEA

Known as German chamomile, *chamomilla* is an antispasmodic and relaxant and used for small children to help ease colic. It is useful for indigestion, IBS, pain, bloating and wind. With a fresh, soothing flavour, it is easy to make and often part of my bedtime ritual as it gives such a gentle soothing.

INGREDIENTS

~ 2 tsp dried chamomile flowers

~ 1 tsp dill fronds

~ 400ml (13fl oz/generous 1½ cups) boiling water

METHOD

Put the fresh and dried herbs in a jug and pour over the boiling water. Leave to steep for 10 minutes, then enjoy.

Storage: Make fresh as required.

Dose: Use as often as you like.

MAKES
About 400 ml
(13fl oz/generous
1½ cups)

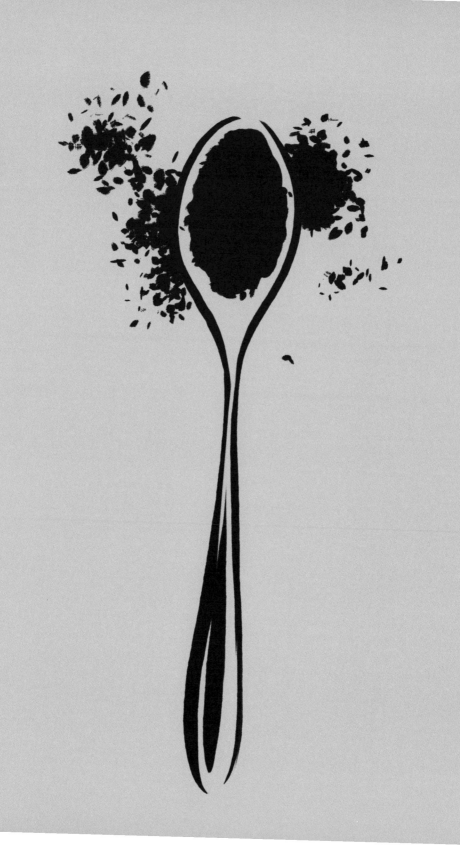

SPOTLIGHT ON
ACTIVATED CHARCOAL

Our ancestors (as well as animals) used charcoal for centuries as a remedy for multiple concerns, due to its unique toxin removing properties. From the Egyptians to the ancient Hindus and Phoenicians it was used to combat intestinal ailments, remove unwanted odours and to purify water long before we rediscovered it in the West.

After a 1963 article in the Journal of Paediatrics resurrected medical interest in charcoal calling it 'the most valuable single agent we possess'. It became more commonly used as a decontaminant after poisoning and its use has increased further in the home, for detoxifying and cleaning.

Activated charcoal was approved by the World Health Organisation in 2019 for the effective treatment of overdoses and poisonings. Made from carbon that has been heated increasing its porosity, activated charcoal is unique for its vast surface area. One teaspoon of the powder has a surface area larger than a football pitch. This means that it can adsorb toxins –removing a soluble substance from a liquid – and bind to many toxins in the gut, reducing their absorption by the body.

Being carbon, charcoal has a positive ionic charge, and most of the toxins and pollutants in our body have a negative charge. They are therefore drawn to the carbon and emitted naturally, before causing any harm. There are no known side effects, carbon is insoluble therefore cannot be digested by the body, so it passes through the system and out leaving no trace.

CHIA & FLAXSEED CONSTIPATION RELIEF SHOT

Bowel movements are so critical to our overall feeling of wellbeing and are a good indication of how healthly we are, so being blocked up is not just uncomfortable, or even painful, but also impacts our general health. Dehydration, lack of fibre and insufficient physical activity can all be contributing factors to a wider cause, which should always be looked at, but you can begin by solving the immediate problem, and adding a shot of these seeds is hugely effective. Laxatives that work to stimulate peristaltic muscle movement are often violent and not useful for long-term use.

INGREDIENTS

~ 1 tbsp chia seeds

~ 1 tbsp flax seeds

~ squeeze of lemon juice

~ 200ml (7fl oz/scant 1 cup) water

METHOD

Put all the ingredients in a glass, stir well and leave for 30 minutes until the seeds look gel-like in consistency. Stir again, then drink immediately.

Storage: Make fresh as required.

Dose: Adults and children over 12 drink 1 serving; children under 12 drink half that quantity.

TIP: If you find the texture unpalatable, blitz up the seeds before mixing with water.

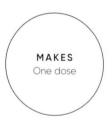

MAKES
One dose

RUNNY HONEY BURN TREATMENT

MAKES
One
application

I would always say it was worth buying the best quality you can with simple ingredients like this for how they will benefit you, but when swiping it over a burn, the last of an older jar will work just as well. It is, as you may imagine by now, the antimicrobial and antiseptic active ingredients that make honey such a healer.

I N G R E D I E N T S ~ 1 tsp raw honey

M E T H O D Using a small knife or wooden lollipop stick, scoop up the honey and apply gently to the burn. Cover with a plaster. **Storage:** Keep honey in an airtight jar in a cool, dark place. **Dose:** Use as required.

SALT WATER & HONEY THROAT GARGLE

MAKES
One
dose

Honey is now the throat hero, so using a concoction to stop infections in their tracks is a great preventative idea. Use this as part of your morning or evening routine.

I N G R E D I E N T S ~ 1 tsp sea salt flakes ~ 200ml (7fl oz/scant 1 cup) warm water ~ 1 tsp raw honey

M E T H O D Mix the ingredients together until dissolved completely. Take a sip and gargle for 10–15 seconds in the back of the throat, with the head back. Spit, then repeat with a fresh mouthful. **Storage:** Make fresh as required. **Dose:** Gargle daily 4–5 times per dose.

CHARCOAL SPLINTER REMOVAL BANDAGE

The charcoal absorption mechanism is useful here in that it can draw splinters out by sitting on the surface.

MAKES
Anough for 4
applications

I N G R E D I E N T S ~ ½ tsp activated charcoal powder ~ 1 tsp coconut oil ~ 1 plaster

M E T H O D Combine the oil with the charcoal and dab a pea-sized amount onto the bandage area of the plaster and apply to the splinter area. Leave on for 12 hours, then change. **Storage:** Keeps for up to a year. **Dose:** Repeat until splinter is out.

TRAVEL

It's no secret that people are ill more often as soon as they leave home, whether that's from new foods, aeroplane travel and increase in contact with possible illness or just giving up their regular routine, suddenly relaxing, or exhaustion and stress. And regular ailments can seem harder to deal with when in unfamiliar climes. There are, however, some ideas I've come across and a handful of things I never leave home without that are natural ways of combatting the most frequent woes of the traveller.

CHARCOAL SICK BUG TONIC

Used in Chinese and Ayurvedic medicine for thousands of years because of its powerful ability to draw toxins and chemicals out of the body, charcoal has been used in the cases of accidental poisonings in the West for a long time, too. When I first mixed this up, I was hoping for a miracle and I got one: a bout of sickness stopped in its tracks. It is now one of my range of remedies on sale – BE SETTLED; we often get asked to send it out by Uber for emergencies.

INGREDIENTS

~ 1 tsp mint leaves

~ 300ml (10½fl oz/1¼ cups) boiling water

~ 1 tsp activated charcoal (use the capsules and pull apart)

MAKES
About 300ml
(10½fl oz/
1¼ cups)

METHOD

Put the mint leaves in a mug and pour over the boiling water. Leave to cool, then strain out the leaves and stir through the activated charcoal. Sip slowly as needed.

Storage: Make fresh as required.

Dose: Use no more than once a day.

NB: It can bind to regular medication, like the contraceptive pill, and other nutrients, so daily use is not advised.

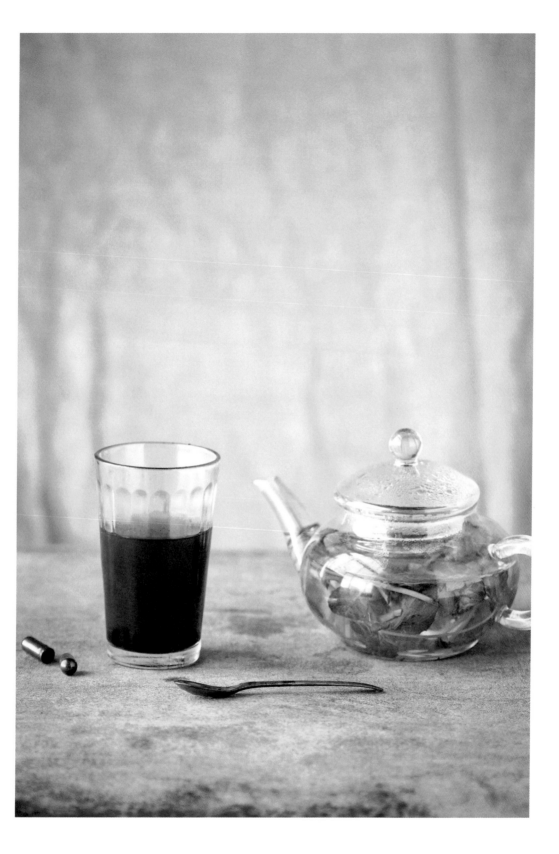

BICARBONATE OF SODA ANTI-ITCH FOR BITES

Another use for this brilliantly multi-dexterous baking staple, the alkaline nature of sodium bicarbonate neutralises the pH of the reddened, infected area and reduces the itching.

INGREDIENTS

~ 1 tbsp bicarbonate of soda (baking soda)

~ about 1 tbsp water

MAKES
One application

METHOD

Put the bicarbonate of soda in a small bowl and gradually add water a drop at a time, mixing until it forms a paste. Apply to the affected areas, leave for 10 minutes, then wash off with water. Repeat as necessary.

Storage: Make fresh as required.

Dose: Use as often as required.

LEMON BALM MOSQUITO REPELLENT

Itchy insect bites and horrible reactions can ruin holidays, particularly for those of us who are susceptible to them – they definitely have their favourites. Lemon balm, a relative of the mint family, is a natural antihistamine that relieves the itch bites can cause. This tonic is a saviour to me, and the bright, summer smell is enough to keep you applying after the itch may have gone.

INGREDIENTS

~ 3 tbsp finely chopped lemon balm leaves

~ 300ml (10½fl oz/scant 1¼ cups) witch hazel (or clear alcohol)

~ 6 drops of lavender essential oil

~ 6 drops of citronella essential oil

~ water

METHOD

Place the leaves in a large glass jar and pour over the witch hazel. Screw on the lid tightly and leave in a dark place for 1–2 weeks.

Drain off and discard the leaves. Pour 100ml (3½fl oz/ scant ½ cup) of the witch hazel into a 200ml (7fl oz/scant 1 cup) spray bottle, then add 2 drops of each of the essential oils and fill up the bottle with water. Shake well to mix. Spray on mosquito bites or any other itchy bites.

Reserve the remaining lemon balm-infused witch hazel and the remaining oils to make 2 more batches.

Storage: Stays fresh in the cupboard for up to 3 months.

Dose: Spray as needed.

TIP: 35–40% budget vodka is ideal instead of witch hazel.

MAKES
About 300ml (10½fl oz/scant 1¼ cups) in three batches

DRY SHAMPOO

In a bind, a dusting of dry shampoo can be a girl's best friend – post-workout, combatting humidity and more. The regular offerings out there can have talc (containing asbestos naturally) and alcohol, which dries the scalp and can harm the hair follicles. This combination, on the other hand, is so simple to put together with pantry staples and can be adapted to any hair colour – using a combo of either cinnamon or cocoa.

INGREDIENTS

~ 2 tbsp arrowroot

~ 1 tbsp ground cinnamon

~ 1 tbsp cocoa (unsweetened chocolate) powder

~ 4 drops of tea tree essential oil (optional)

METHOD

Mix all the ingredients together in a bowl, including the tea tree oil, if using. Funnel into a jar. Apply with a powder brush to the roots.

Storage: Keeps fresh for up to a year.

Dose: Use as needed.

MAKES
About 125g
(4½oz)

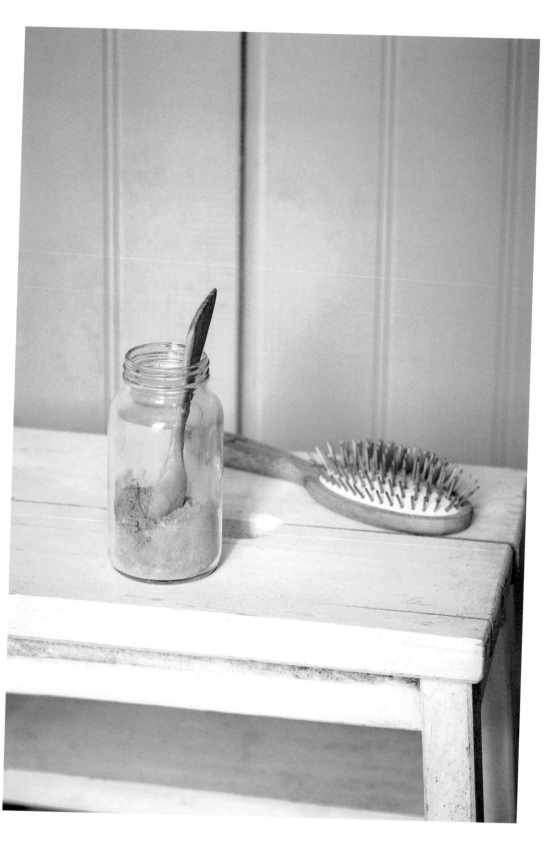

AFTER SUN SOOTHING SPRITZ

Burnt or just feeling sun overload, your thirsty summer skin will love this hydrating mist, which includes all the skin-calming favourites from the aloe vera plant to chamomile, reducing redness, easing the inflammation and soothing the pain.

INGREDIENTS

~ 2 tsp dried chamomile

~ 200ml (7fl oz/scant 1 cup) boiling water

~ 3 tbsp aloe vera gel

~ 5 drops of lavender essential oil

METHOD

Add the chamomile to the boiling water and leave to steep for 10 minutes.

Drain and reserve the liquid, leaving it to cool fully.

Combine all the ingredients and use a spray bottle to mist over the skin as needed.

Storage: Keeps fresh for up to 1 month.

Dose: Apply liberally.

MAKES
About 250ml
(8fl oz/1 cup)

HEAT RASH & SUNBURN RELIEF MILK

Over-exposure to UV rays causes inflammation and pain to the skin, so cooling it as well as reducing the inflammation is the most effective way to soothe. Drinking more water is also useful, as sunburn can draw liquid from the skin to heal.

INGREDIENTS

~ 1 aloe vera leaf, split in half
(or pure aloe vera gel)
~ coconut oil

METHOD

Smooth the aloe vera onto the affected areas and leave to dry. Alternate with the moisturising coconut oil for a combined, natural approach.

Storage: Make fresh as required.

Dose: Use generously and frequently.

MAKES
One
application

SPOTLIGHT ON
YOUR EVERYDAY IMPACT

With a planet in undoubted crisis, ever-increasing global temperatures, countless species under threat of extinction, the deterioration of the health of our oceans and swathes of forest land being wiped out every day, our impact on the Earth has never been more critical. The human imprint on nature's ecosystem is evident as everything becomes more out of balance in our post-industrial, profit-focused and consumer-driven world.

As individuals, the instinct to assume no responsibility is tempting – so huge is the task and so seemingly meaningless our personal impact. But we can make changes, however small, because together we can have an impact that will turn things around.

Renowned British naturalist David Attenborough has spent a lifetime rallying support for the preservation of our planet. Despite the damage that continues to be done, he insists that it is never too late to help, and we are never too small to make a difference.

As consumers, we can make a lasting impact with our everyday choices. By using natural ingredients, and not those with commercially derived materials, we are bypassing industrial production and transportation as well as the chemical fallout of what lands in our water system. We are also preventing unwanted ingredients from getting into our bodies and affecting our health, short or long term.

A NOTE ON MICROPLASTICS

Preservatives, perfumes and microplastics are all in over-supply in many commercial beauty, cleaning and household products, so we are breathing them in and absorbing them through our skin.

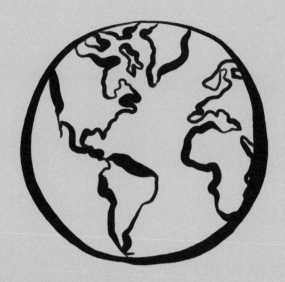

So miniscule they can find their way into our blood stream, and throughout our systems, each type of plastic can contain thousands of additives and chemicals that then leach into the surrounding air and water cycle.

The scourge of these miniscule particles is staggering. UK researchers have recently discovered microplastics in breast milk, deep within the lungs and in the blood of donors for the first time, in four out of five fish tested in New Zealand, in our deepest oceans and on the top of Mount Everest. Experiments have already demonstrated the effect of microplastics on human health – causing both allergic reactions and cell death – and clinical research continues.

But we cannot sit back and wait for science and data-collection to come up with resolute strategies; we need to act now. Keeping the products in our homes free from these seems to be by far the most forward-thinking approach.

The head of the American Lung Association likened the microplastics discussion to the smoking debate of last century: 'Will we find out in 40 years that microplastics in the lungs led to premature ageing of the lung or to emphysema? We don't know.' In the meantime, avoiding them is not going to do any harm to us, our waterways or our wildlife.

ACKNOWLEDGEMENTS

Thank you to everyone who willed this book into existence. The fabulous lot from my blog who made all the remedies and told me how much you loved them. Bettina, our chance meeting that rainy night in Old Street, and your enthusiasm gave me the dream publisher. Thanks Kate for being cool and assembling a crack team of talent to create beauty as promised. Julia's design. Nass and Rachel for some dreamy shoot days, making magic.

To my friends who I haven't seen enough of recently, and those who I have and have been tireless testers and readers and style aficionados. Trans-Atlantic creative dream team, Lisa and Tom, dialling in their very best from LA – you are loved.

Charlotte, for knowing and giving so much.

Running my remedies business whilst writing was only possible because of my right-hand and wing commander, Jo: thank you for never questioning and always having more steam.

My sister Lou, for making our writing retreat in the hills so perfect. There would be no book if there had been no space or time or quiet in your home in which to write it.

Thank you Mum and Dad, for opening the world up.

And to my home team: Robin, Jethro, Calypso and Phoenix, who were the why. Thank you for eating, sipping, nodding and cheering me on with passion all these years.

ABOUT THE AUTHOR

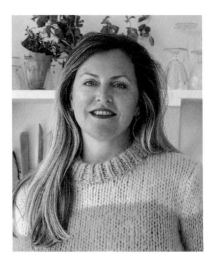

Lizzie King is a mother of three, nutritional health coach, author of *Lizzie Loves Healthy Family Food*, founder of award-winning natural remedies' company 'Lizzie Loves Nature's Botanicals' and the popular food blog, Lizzie Loves Healthy. Lizzie began her career in film and the *Harry Potter* franchise, then switched focus to nutrition and food after starting her family, and has been creating recipes and remedies to keep them in the best health for the last 15 years. She lives in West London with her husband, three children, a golden retriever and two cats.
www.lizzie-loves.com / **@lizzieloveshealthy**

INDEX

A NOTE ON INGREDIENTS

While these recipes use natural ingredients, have been exhaustively tested and are suitable for the vast

majority of people, those with skin allergies or very sensitive skin should patch test body products to check

for a reaction. Neither the author, the publisher nor anyone connected with the production of this book can

be held responsible for any issues arising out of the use or misuse of the information provided.

Published in 2023 by OH Editions,
part of Welbeck Publishing Group.
Offices in: London – 20 Mortimer Street, London W1T 3JW &
Sydney – 205 Commonwealth Street, Surry Hills 2010
www.welbeckpublishing.com

Design and layout © 2023 OH Editions
Text copyright © 2023 Lizzie King
Photography © Nassima Rothacker
Illustrations © 2023 Julia Murray

Lizzie King has asserted her moral rights to be identified as the author of this Work in accordance
with the Copyright Designs and Patents Act 1988.

All rights reserved. No part of this publication may be reproduced, stored in a retrieval system, or
transmitted in any form or by any means, electronically, mechanically, by photocopying, recording or
otherwise, without the prior permission of the copyright owners and the publishers.

A CIP catalogue record for this book is available from the British Library.

ISBN 978-1-80453-052-8

Publisher: Kate Pollard
Desk Editor: Matt Tomlinson
Photographer: Nassima Rothacker
Food and prop stylist: Rachel De Thample
Editor: Wendy Hobson
Designer: Julia Murray and Steven Ranson
Indexer: Cathy Heath
Production controller: Arlene Alexander
Colour reproduction: P2D

Printed and bound by Leo in China

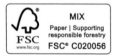

MIX
Paper | Supporting
responsible forestry
FSC® C020056

10 9 8 7 6 5 4 3 2 1

Disclaimer:
Any names, characters, trademarks, service marks and trade names detailed in this book is the
property of their respective owners and are used solely for identification and reference purposes. This
book is a publication of OH Editions, part of Welbeck Publishing Group and has not been licensed,
approved, sponsored or endorsed by any person or entity.